SIMULATION SCENARIOS FOR NURSING EDUCATION

TAMMY J. HALE

PATRICIA M. AHLSCHLAGER

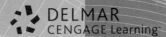

DELMAR
CENGAGE Learning

Australia • Brazil • Japan • Korea • Mexico • Singapore • Spain • United Kingdom • United States

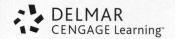

Simulation Scenarios for Nursing Education, 1st Edition
Tammy J. Hale, Patricia M. Ahlschlager

Vice President, Career and Professional Editorial: Dave Garza

Director of Learning Solutions: Matt Kane

Executive Editor: Steven Helba

Managing Editor: Marah Bellegarde

Senior Product Manager: Juliet Steiner

Editorial Assistant: Meghan E. Orvis

Vice President, Career and Professional Marketing: Jennifer Ann Baker

Marketing Director: Wendy Mapstone

Senior Marketing Manager: Michele McTighe

Marketing Coordinator: Scott Chrysler

Production Director: Carolyn Miller

Production Manager: Andrew Crouth

Senior Content Project Manager: Jim Zayicek

Senior Art Director: Jack Pendleton

For product information and technology assistance, contact us at
Cengage Learning Customer & Sales Support, 1-800-354-9706

For permission to use material from this text or product,
submit all requests online at **www.cengage.com/permissions**.
Further permissions questions can be e-mailed to
permissionrequest@cengage.com

Library of Congress Control Number: 2010920722

ISBN-13: 978-1-4354-8413-9

ISBN-10: 1-4354-8413-4

Delmar
5 Maxwell Drive
Clifton Park, NY 12065-2919
USA

Cengage Learning is a leading provider of customized learning solutions with office locations around the globe, including Singapore, the United Kingdom, Australia, Mexico, Brazil, and Japan. Locate your local office at: **international.cengage.com/region**

Cengage Learning products are represented in Canada by Nelson Education, Ltd.

To learn more about Delmar, visit **www.cengage.com/delmar**

Purchase any of our products at your local college store or at our preferred online store **www.CengageBrain.com**

1 2 3 4 5 6 7 13 12 11 10

Contents

Dedication

To Todd, Isaac, and Ellie. Your love and support continually inspire and energize me. To my mother and father for providing me a solid foundation and continued encouragement. To Michelle Sundby for providing my children nurturing care while I am away from them, you truly are a blessing. Last but not least to Pat, a great friend who embarked on this adventure with me.

Tammy

In memory of my mother Jean Hafner, whose career as a nurse inspired me. To my dear husband, your support is without limits. For all my family who encouraged us. Special thanks to Tammy Hale, who was the inspiration and driving force to complete this project.

Patricia

Preface

Simulation Scenarios for Nursing Education

Simulation Scenarios for Nursing Education is a valuable resource that can contribute to students' success in achieving the learning outcomes related to participation in simulation scenarios. The dynamic scenarios in this resource will provide students with a variety of educational opportunities to further develop essential nursing skills. Research supports active learning using simulation in education. When comparing simulation with written case studies, Leigh (2008) stated, "Students participating in HPS (human patient simulator) had a greater sense of involvement with diverse learning; valued the educational experience; and perceived the active learning, support, objectives, feedback and fidelity as being more significant. . ." (page 6). Simulation allows students the chance to conceptualize difficult concepts while practicing in a safe learning environment.

We value the active and unique learning experiences that simulation can provide and have witnessed first-hand how students have excelled during scenario events. As educators we use simulation frequently and fully understand the importance of student preparation, which is vital to accomplishment of the simulation goals. When students have the chance to read the goals and outcomes, patient information, and guidelines for preparation prior to the simulation experience, they are able to enhance their performance. This text will provide important information for students to review as they prepare for the assigned simulation scenario.

A unique feature of this resource is the inclusion of scenarios for both the practical nursing student and the registered nursing student. Combining both levels of practice provides an option for the continued use of the text for students who choose to further their education past a practical nursing diploma/degree. Conducting simulations with both practical nursing and registered nursing students is possible because all students will have access to simulation information within the student resource.

Organization

Simulation Scenarios for Nursing Education begins with an introductory chapter that provides a substantial amount of information with clear guidelines to students. The first chapter describes simulation, its benefits in education, the importance of preparation, student roles, and how to communicate as a team. In addition, the first chapter explains the general principles of how a simulation scenario will progress, the evaluation (grading) process, and a list of helpful hints.

Following Chapter 1, the book is divided into two sections: Simulation Scenarios for Practical/Vocational Nursing Students and Simulation Scenarios for Registered Nursing Students. The scenarios provided in each of these sections are similar in nature, but the written details account for the differing scope of practice. Educators are welcome to use the scenarios with only the student group for which they are written, or conduct joint simulation experiences with practical nursing students and registered nursing students together. The outline of scenarios that follows applies to both sections of this resource.

The simulation scenarios are designed for teams of four students. Designated student roles include data collection/assessment, medication administration, team leader/supervisor, and family member. General concepts for each team member are outlined in Chapter 1. Subsequent chapters further elaborate on specific considerations for each student role. Students should review the guidelines in Chapter 1 as well as in each chapter as they prepare for simulation events.

Most simulation scenarios are also constructed with a patient chart, physician orders, and a medication administration record (MAR). Students should review the patient chart during the simulation because this resource will further assist with simulated patient care. Please note that a few simulation scenarios do not contain all information when the patient is presenting to a clinic or emergency department. This is intentional because these scenarios are intended to provide a greater challenge to the students.

Features

1. Chapter 1 clearly outlines the basic principles of the simulation experience. It introduces students to the value of simulation exercises, orients them to student roles, explains the progression of simulation events, and provides helpful hints for success.
2. Ten pre-written scenarios (seven adult and three pediatric) provide an enriched learning experience for students.

3. Each student scenario includes goals/outcomes, patient information, guidelines for preparation, and a corresponding case study for each exercise.

4. Case studies are provided with each scenario to further encourage student critical thinking on the designated topic.

About the Authors

Tammy Hale, BSN, RN

Ms. Hale graduated from the University of North Dakota in 1998. Her work experience has been primarily in the emergency department. Currently she is nursing faculty at Minnesota State Community and Technical College in Wadena, Minnesota. She is a graduate student at Minnesota State University Moorhead pursuing a master's degree in nursing education.

Patricia Ahlschlager, MSN, RN

Ms. Ahlschlager graduated from Rapid City Regional diploma nursing program in 1976, Metropolitan State College in Denver, and Minnesota State University Moorhead with a master's degree in nurse education. Her work experience has included medical surgical, intensive care, supervision, and home care. Currently she is on the nursing faculty at Minnesota State Community and Technical College in Wadena, Minnesota.

Acknowledgments

Although many individuals have helped us in our journey to bring this text to publication, we would like to acknowledge the following individuals in particular.

We would like to acknowledge our students who energize and inspire us daily. We look forward to teaching those so willing to enter the nursing profession. May you find success in all that you do!

To the faculty and staff at Minnesota State Community and Technical College–Wadena campus who make our time at work enjoyable. A special thank you to Dave Uselman, Misty Wilkie-Condiff, Karoline Bagent, Sara Erickson, Susan Seaborn, Nancy Krause, Sonja Amundson, Karen Treangen, and Bill Evans. Your support and encouragement is appreciated. We would also like to thank our campus administration for granting permission to include pictures of our simulation lab within this text.

We thank Sharyl Rinkel and Kathy Kleen at Tri-County Hospital in Wadena, Minnesota, for providing us with a variety of resources. Your continued support does not go unnoticed.

Reviewers

Marylee Bressie, RN, CCRN, CCNS, CEN,
  BC-CVN II, MSN
Instructor
Division of Nursing Adult Health
Spring Hill College
Mobile, Alabama

Doreen DeAngelis
Nursing Instructor
Pennsylvania State University at Fayette
Uniontown, West Virginia

Pamela "Penni" Ellis, RN, MSN
Nursing Faculty
Mohave Community College
Bullhead City, Arizona

Jaclynn A. Johnson, RNC-OB, MSN
Freshman Lead Instructor
Otero Junior College
La Junta, Colorado

Gary Laustsen, PhD, FNP-BC
Assistant Professor
Director of Simulation
Oregon Health and Science University
La Grande, Oregon

Jodelle Lee, RN, BSN
Simulation Manager
Bohecker College
Columbus, Ohio

Denise Root, RN, MSN
Nursing Department Director
Otero Junior College
La Junta, Colorado

Donna C. Semar, RN, PhD
Coordinator
Steele Innovation Learning Center
University of Arizona
College of Nursing
Tucson, Arizona

Kimberly Valich, RN, MSN
Nursing Faculty and Department
  Chairperson
South Suburban College
South Holland, Illinois

Welcome to Simulation

This chapter will introduce you to simulation and provide you with information on how to prepare for each scenario. Simulation is a method of learning that enables students to provide nursing care to a human patient simulator (HPS), a life-like mannequin. An HPS may be able to replicate patient data such as heart sounds, lung sounds, bowel sounds, and vocal sounds. The HPS is used within a simulation environment designed to represent an actual clinical setting. During the simulation scenario, nursing students are expected to demonstrate competence in (a) nursing assessment, (b) practical skills, (c) communication, (d) safe nursing care, and (e) the ability to function as part of a healthcare team.

As a student, you may not have opportunities to care for patients with different diagnostic categories during your scheduled clinical rotations. Simulation helps to bridge the potential gap in knowledge that results from differing opportunities available to students. Scenarios are designed to teach specific learning objectives that incorporate the nursing process and skill competencies. In the clinical setting students typically take on an observation role when working with patients who are critically ill. Simulation allows you the opportunity to actively provide nursing care to a variety of patients within a safe learning environment. Many people are satisfied with this method of instruction because it allows students the ability to work within a team to learn necessary skills to provide patient care. We believe simulation will better prepare you for your role in the nursing profession.

Simulation Preparation

Thorough preparation is essential for simulation success and cannot be overemphasized. Each student should review all possible assigned roles. Well-prepared teams achieve higher grades. The chapters within this text will provide students with specific information to review prior to each simulation scenario. The typical time allotted for each simulation exercise is 20–30 minutes. Students will have minimal time to look up information during the simulation. The amount of time needed to prepare will vary. Students may consider preparing as a team so that they can assist each other in the comprehension of difficult topics.

Team preparation should begin by discussing the patient history in full detail; be sure that you fully understand the medical conditions presented. Students must then review all medications and note (a) the medication indications, (b) various available routes, (c) potential side effects, (d) safe dosages (especially in pediatric simulations), and (e) methods for evaluating the medication's effectiveness. Skills listed within the simulation chapter should be reviewed. Preparation for nursing skills should involve consideration of all patient aspects (e.g., male versus female, pediatric versus adult). Carefully review all information presented within the assigned chapter. Evaluation is expected after the performance of all nursing interventions. Students should evaluate if the intervention performed resulted in a positive or negative HPS response and implement further interventions as needed.

The educator will provide an orientation to the simulation environment and the HPS. Basic knowledge of equipment location and HPS capabilities will be beneficial during all simulation experiences. If the performance of a particular skill (e.g., urinary catheter insertion) is anticipated, the necessary supplies should be located during orientation. Additionally, students should practice and pre-plan the performance of this skill. All simulation scenarios will require students to manually obtain vital signs. Practice obtaining vital signs on the designated HPS prior to the simulation scenario will help with accuracy.

Student Roles during Simulation

The assigned student roles within the simulation scenarios are listed in the following sections. Students should be familiar with all roles because they hold equal importance. Though the simulation exercise may be graded on a team basis, the educator may reserve the right to award different points to various team members based on performance. Students are encouraged to assist one another because the experience is a team effort. In the event a fellow teammate is having difficulty moving ahead, other members should be prepared to provide assistance. At the discretion of the educator roles can be combined, deleted, or added.

RN Student Roles

The suggested RN student roles of supervisor, medication nurse, assessment nurse, family member, and fifth student are discussed in detail in the following section. Students should thoroughly review each role and prepare to perform the duties of all roles. In the event that PN students will comprise some of the team members, the PN roles should also be reviewed.

Supervisor

The supervisor oversees and directs the progress of the team. Designated duties include double-checking medications and dosage calculations, assisting with assessment, double-checking vital signs to ensure accuracy, and providing patient/family member education. The supervisor will be required to notify the health care provider as the patient's condition warrants. The supervisor may consult other team members as questions arise. The supervisor must demonstrate leadership. Coordination of the team effort and accurate reporting to a primary health care provider (e.g., physician or advanced practice nurse) is expected. Delegation is a key component of this leadership role.

Medication Nurse

This student will review the patient chart and ordered medications and treatments. The team member's responsibility is the administration of ordered medications. In the event that new orders are received, this member must ensure that the orders are written by the supervisor who obtained the orders. Following the administration of medications, this team member must document the administration on the provided medication administration record (MAR). This student may consult other team members if questions arise. The student should be sure to note all the medication "rights": (a) right medication (know brand/generic names), (b) right dose (is this a safe dose), (c) right route, (d) right time (check last dose if PRN), (e) right patient (check the name band and two identifiers), and (f) right documentation of medication administration. When applicable, students must also consider the rate of the medication administration, which is especially important with intravenous (IV) push medications. Students must be sure to state out loud the dosage being administered (e.g., 2 mL or 2 tablets), which is done to assist the educator with grading. Dosage calculations will be required. Patient education in relation to medication is expected. Evaluation of all medication actions related to the scenario is necessary. For example, if acetaminophen is administered for a fever, students should recheck the patient's temperature. Other points to consider include expiration date, allergies, and whether a pre-administration blood pressure or pulse is needed.

Assessment Nurse

This student must conduct a thorough head-to-toe assessment and communicate with team members any abnormalities observed during the assessment. For example, relay to the medication nurse an abnormal blood pressure, as this information may be important to note when administering antihypertensives. Once the assessment is complete, this student should perform skills and procedures that are ordered by the health care provider. The student may need to demonstrate prioritization of the assessment and skills. A patient displaying respiratory compromise may need interventions such as oxygen application prior to listening to bowel sounds. The student may receive help from other students at any time.

Family Member

It is the role of the family member to provide the patient history and advocate for the patient. Unless five team members are present, the family member may record information obtained, such as vital signs, for charting exercises. This student may also prompt teammates to gather assessment data, give a medication, or perform a certain task through questions that a family member might ask. For example, if the student observes that the temperature has not yet been obtained, a comment such as "I'm curious to know his temperature" may be appropriate. The student assigned the role of the family member is encouraged to be creative. The family member may choose to hug, kiss, hold hands with, or provide comfort to the HPS.

Fifth Student

In the event that a team of five students is assigned, the fifth student may be responsible for documenting the simulation events. This student must follow the format outlined by the educator. The fifth student may also assist with ordered procedures and provide a verbal report upon the conclusion of the simulation exercise.

PN Student Roles

The suggested PN student roles of team leader, medication nurse, data collection nurse, family member, and fifth student are discussed in detail in the following section. Students should thoroughly review each role and prepare to perform the duties of all roles. In the event that RN students will comprise some of the team members, the RN roles should also be reviewed.

Team Leader

The team leader provides guidance to fellow teammates during the simulation exercise. Designated duties include double-checking medications and dosage calculations, assisting with data collection, double-checking vital signs to ensure accuracy, and providing the patient/family information regarding the plan of care. The team leader will be required to notify the nursing supervisor as the patient's condition warrants. The team leader may consult other team members as questions arise.

Medication Nurse

This student will review the patient chart and ordered medications and treatments. The administration of ordered medications is this team member's responsibility. Following the administration of medications, this team member must document the administration on the provided medication administration record (MAR). This student may consult other team members if questions arise. The student should be sure to note all the medication "rights": (a) right medication (know brand/generic names), (b) right dose (is this a safe dose), (c) right route, (d) right time (check last dose if PRN), (e) right patient (check the name band and two identifiers), and (f) right documentation of medication administration. When applicable, students must also consider the rate of the medication administration; this is especially important with IV piggyback medications. Students must be sure to state out loud the dosage being administered (e.g., 2 mL or 2 tablets), which is done to assist the educator with grading. Dosage calculations will be required. Patient education in relation to medication is expected. Evaluation of all medication actions related to the scenario is necessary. For example, if acetaminophen is administered for a fever, students should recheck the patient's temperature. Other points to consider include expiration date, allergies, and whether a pre-administration blood pressure or pulse is needed.

Data Collection Nurse

This student must collect data pertinent to the patient's condition and communicate with team members any abnormalities observed. For example, relay to the medication nurse an abnormal blood pressure because this information may be important to note when administering antihypertensives. Once data collection is complete, this student should perform skills and procedures that are ordered by the primary care provider. The student may need to demonstrate prioritization of data collection and skills. For example, a patient displaying respiratory compromise may need interventions such as oxygen application prior to listening to bowel sounds. This student may receive help from other students at any time.

Family Member

It is the role of the family member to provide the patient history and advocate for the patient. Unless five team members are present, the family member may record information obtained for charting exercises such as vital signs. The student may also prompt teammates to gather data, give a medication, or perform a certain task through questions that a family member might ask. For example, if the student observes that the temperature has not yet been obtained, a comment such as "I'm curious to know his temperature" may be appropriate. The student assigned the role of the family member is encouraged to be creative. The family member may choose to hug, kiss, hold hands with, or provide comfort to the HPS.

Fifth Student

In the event that a team of five students is assigned, the fifth student may be responsible for documenting the simulation events. This student must follow the format outlined by the educator. The fifth student may also assist with ordered procedures and provide a verbal report upon the conclusion of the simulation exercise.

Communication

Communication among team members during the simulation scenario is important. Errors made may affect the overall team grade. Students who observe errors within the simulation exercise are encouraged to speak up. For example, if a student contaminates a sterile field, a verbal cue to correct the contamination should be provided. Uncorrected errors may result in a significant point reduction. It is imperative that team members express concerns in a professional, non-demeaning way. Team members should then consult with each other to provide an appropriate suggestion for error correction.

Simulation Supplies

The following list of standard simulation supplies may be available for students to use. Please note that there may be slight variations amid simulation environments. During the simulation exercise, if you feel that a required supply is missing, speak up and verbally discuss appropriate actions to take.

- A sample patient chart for each simulation exercise. Students should be sure to review the chart contents. No access to the chart will be permitted prior to the simulation exercise.
- The human patient simulator with proper identification (i.e., name band) in a patient care environment. Figure 1-1 is an example of a simulated patient care environment (from the Minnesota State Community and Technical College nursing simulation lab in Wadena, Minnesota).
- Oxygen equipment—Adult and pediatric nasal cannulas, simple masks, non-rebreathers, bag valve masks (ambu bags), and nebulizer supplies. A nebulizer machine may be used within the simulation. A wall

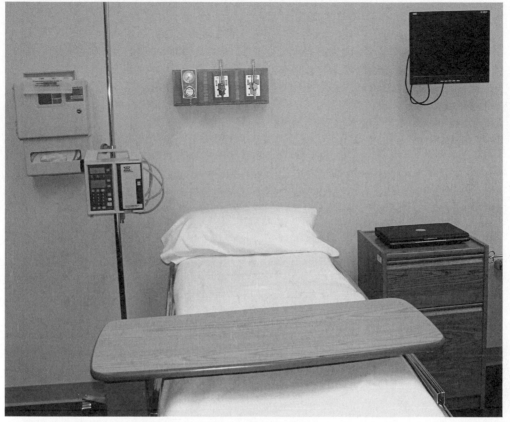

Courtesy of Delmer Cengage Learning.

FIGURE 1-1 **Simulated single-patient care environment**

mount unit containing a suction, oxygen, and air may also be available. Figure 1-2 is an example of a wall mount unit.

■ An incentive spirometer (IS) should be available.

■ Vital sign apparatuses—Standard adult and pediatric blood pressure cuffs (note that some HPSs require that you use particular equipment), tympanic and oral thermometers, oxygen saturation monitor, and four to five stethoscopes.

■ Pain scale—Both adult and pediatric versions. A behavior pain scale, numeric pain scale, and Wong-Baker Faces Scale may be available.

■ IV supplies—Primary and secondary tubing, IV start kits, a variety of IV cannulas (24, 22, 20, and 18 gauge). Students may be required to use smaller gauges to preserve the simulator. However, students should state which size is appropriate for the situation. An IV pump may also be made available. IV fluids will be provided when necessary. Please note that infusion of IV fluids into the HPS may cause damage; consult the educator for further guidelines. Figure 1-3 shows an example of an IV supply drawer.

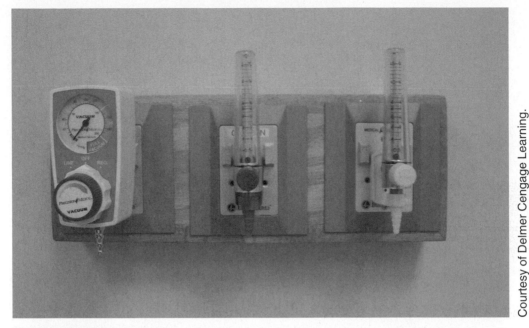

Courtesy of Delmer Cengage Learning.

FIGURE 1-2 Wall mount unit

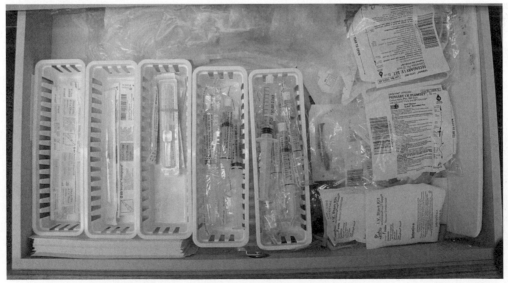

Courtesy of Delmer Cengage Learning.

FIGURE 1-3 IV supply drawer

■ Medication cart—Simulated medications will be available. Be sure to check the medication label prior to administration.

■ Telemetry monitor—Students should understand how to apply a five-lead telemetry monitor. The student may be required to obtain one set of manual vital signs prior to application of an automated blood pressure cuff and telemetry monitor.

- Suction supplies—Appropriate suction apparatus should be attached to a wall mount unit. Sterile suction supplies, appropriate tubing, and a Yankauer suction tip may be available for students to use. Because the wall mount suction device may not be fully functioning, a portable suction unit may be used in the event that actual demonstration of suction is required.
- Nasogastric (NG) supplies—Various NG tube sizes and irrigation supplies, including connectors, NG taping devices, and a safety pin. A gastrostomy tube (G-tube) and 60 mL syringe are also necessary.
- Dressing supplies—2 × 2's, 4 × 4's, bandage wraps, ACE wraps (elastic bandages) of various sizes, abdominal dressing pads, tape, a transparent dressing, and a wound measuring device.
- Gloves—Various sizes of non-sterile and sterile gloves. Be sure to inform the educator if you are allergic to latex products.
- Personal Protective Equipment (PPE)—Gowns, goggles, and masks.
- Sterile saline bottles.
- Syringes—Various intramuscular (IM), subcutaneous (SubQ), and intradermal (ID) syringes and needles may be available. Alcohol prep pads and syringes without may be available as well. Note the location of the sharps container in the simulation room prior to the beginning of the simulation.
- Catheters—Indwelling catheter kits and mini catheter kits. Both adult and pediatric sizes may be included.
- Blood glucose monitors—Capillary blood glucose monitor with lancets and strips. A carbohydrate counting reference guide may also be available.
- Standard patient care supplies—Emesis basin, items to provide oral hygiene, water pitcher, and cup. Bed linens, pillows, towels, washcloths, and diapers for the infant HPS.
- Miscellaneous supplies—Pen light, Glasgow Coma Scale, and a telephone.

Simulation Scenario

At the start of the simulation scenario the educator may decide to assign team members their specific roles. The team of students will then perform the beginning steps. Students should spend less than five minutes completing the beginning steps (washing hands, introducing self to patients, and checking the name band). Next, team members should begin to complete their individual assigned tasks. The student assigned to the assessment/data collection role should begin gathering patient data. If a concerning observation is discovered, the information should be relayed to fellow teammates. At this time, the student assigned the role of the medication nurse should begin reviewing the primary care provider's orders and begin preparing necessary medications. The student assigned the role of family member should be continually interacting with fellow teammates, providing outlined information obtained within the text. The student assigned the role of supervisor/team leader should assume a leadership role directing all team members. Specific guidelines for each student role will be provided in each chapter.

Grading of Simulation Scenarios

The educator will provide students information related to grade construction. Each chapter within this text contains an outline of recommended grading guidelines. The components of grading may include (a) beginning steps, (b) assessment/data collection, (c) implementation, (d) evaluation, (e) verbal report, and (f) student professionalism. Students should work together as a team, guiding each other and demonstrating cooperation. Students who work well as a team tend to perform better in simulation exercises and may earn a higher score as a result.

Students should remain professional during the simulation scenario because it constitutes a portion of the grade. Prior to entering the simulation environment, students should evaluate adherence to the dress code as discussed by faculty. If a member of the team is in violation of the dress code, it may affect the overall team grade. As stated previously, students should verbally address any observed mistakes and express the appropriate action to implement as a result. All members of the team are expected to participate equally. Allowing one member of the team to dominate the simulation scenario should be avoided.

Confidentiality

Simulation confidentiality cannot be stressed enough. Teams that have completed the simulation exercise must avoid sharing information with teams who have yet to complete the experience. Confidentiality is an ethical responsibility required of all nursing professionals. The simulation exercise allows students to practice confidentiality. Significant point reduction in the overall simulation grade may result if a breech in confidentiality occurs. Students may want to reflect on the fact that teams who have been provided information regarding the simulation experience typically outperform the previous teams who supplied the "answers." If subsequent simulation teams outperform previous teams, it may cause the educator to question why previous teams were insufficiently prepared.

Debriefing

Debriefing occurs upon the conclusion of the simulation exercise and allows for review of the simulation events. The debriefing process will be guided by the educator and should reflect on the positive and negative aspects that occurred. The debriefing process is vital and enhances the students' comprehension of desired learning objectives. Components of the debriefing process vary but may include verbal reflection and/or review of audiovisual recordings. Students should not feel threatened during this process and should not attack other students or make negative comments. The simulation experience should end on a positive note. The debriefing should help you understand how each action of the team is crucial to ensure safe patient care. Educators have found that this time with students after the conclusion of the simulation allows the most learning to occur. Addressing mistakes that are made during the simulation exercise can potentially decrease the likelihood that students will repeat the same mistakes in a clinical setting. Students have shared repeatedly that the simulation experience has been helpful for them when they are in a clinical situation similar to the scenarios. Safety is component emphasized in the debriefing to provide further guidelines for each student to carry into his or her practice. Debriefing allows the student to engage in open verbal exchange to evaluate the simulation performance and learn further.

Additional Hints

Review the following helpful hints to assist you in preparing for each simulation scenario.

- Pre-steps to patient care include proper washing of hands, introducing yourself to the patient, establishing patient identification via two identifiers (e.g., name and date of birth), providing privacy, and using gloves and personal protective equipment (PPE) when necessary.
- Fully review the assessment/data collection process.
- Recall each step of the nursing process while participating in simulation scenarios.
- Every simulation exercise will require students to demonstrate how to manually obtain all patient vital signs including blood pressure, apical pulse, respirations, oxygen saturation, and temperature. Understand how the HPS functions to increase competency of these skills. Because accuracy is important, a team member may wish to recheck vital signs.
- Be familiar with all HPS functions. Know what the HPS can do. Some models allow students to auscultate lung sounds, heart sounds, bowel sounds, and a blood pressure.

- Use therapeutic communication with the HPS and family member during the simulation exercise.
- Educate the HPS/family member about the medications being administered and procedures being performed during the exercise. Provide education on the medical condition as time allows. Never miss an opportunity to educate the patient/family in the scenario.
- Review dosage calculations. Understand how to calculate medication dosages based on weight and how to calculate the rate of intravenous (IV) fluid infusion.
- Document all administered medications on the medication administration record (MAR). Because the educator may require the simulation event to be documented, record simulation information for later use in the form of a nurse's note.
- RN students should be prepared to provide a verbal report to the primary health care provider and receive verbal orders via phone.
- PN students should be prepared to report changes in patient condition to the RN supervisor.
- Review where simulation supplies are located.
- Outlined dress codes must be adhered to during the simulation exercise. If a fellow student is observed not adhering to the guidelines, be sure to address the issue prior to the exercise as this may affect the overall team grade.
- Help each other. If a fellow student is having difficulties, assist him/her. Remember that this is a team effort. Allowing a fellow student to struggle may result in a lower overall grade for the team.
- Talk to the HPS as a "real" patient. Ask him/her questions; the educator will provide the verbal response.
- Explain the plan of care to the HPS/family member and keep them informed.
- *Always remember safety!* Be sure to check ID bands, wash hands, and double-check dosage calculations. Do not take shortcuts during the simulation exercise. If a fellow teammate is observed jeopardizing patient safety, speak up and correct the incident.
- Effective communication among team members, with the HPS, and with other health care providers is vital. At times, communicating may prove to be the most challenging aspect of the simulation exercise.
- Do not share information with teams that have not yet completed the simulation exercise because it may negatively impact your grade.
- Be advised that the educator will not guide the team during the simulation. Simulation is a safe environment for students to demonstrate nursing skills independent of the educator's instruction.
- Students may prepare for the simulation exercise by reviewing various sources of information including nursing textbooks, nursing journals,

and the Internet. Locate key terms in the provided scenario to assist with data searches. Web references are not included in this publication due to their changing nature. The preferred resources to use when studying are nursing textbooks and medical search engines.

- ■ Enjoy the learning process. Eagerly explore the presented concepts, realizing that the information and skills you gain will assist in providing quality patient care.

Final Note

Simulations assist students to gain factual knowledge, principles, and skills they can apply in the professional setting. By participating in simulation, you will learn to make decisions and evaluate the consequences of those decisions. This active participation is useful to achieve pre-set learning objectives. The authors of this text wish you well in your future simulation experiences.

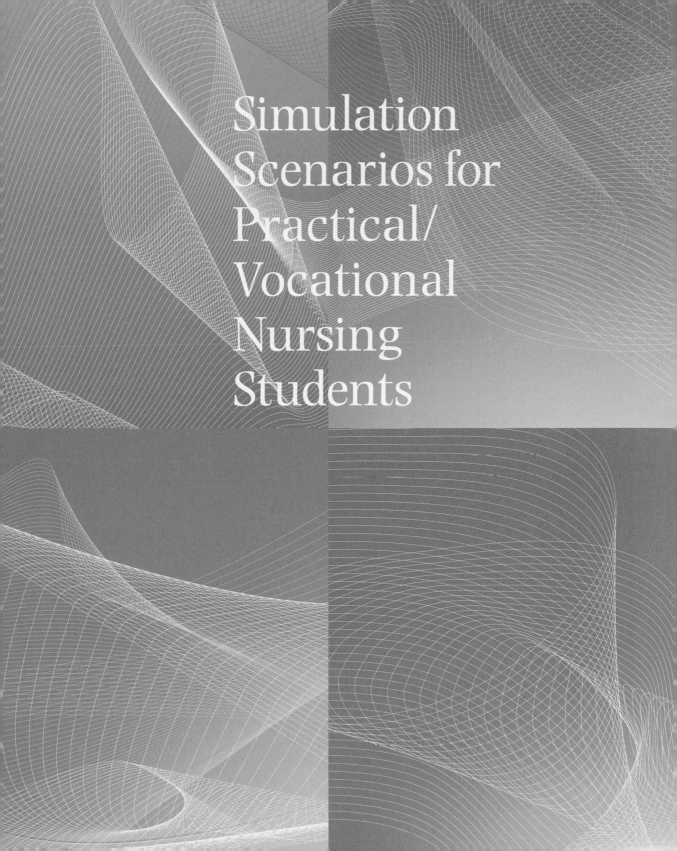

Simulation Scenarios for Practical/ Vocational Nursing Students

Data Collection & Medication Administration (Adult)

Goals/Outcomes of Simulation Exercise

- Students will demonstrate data collection and identify abnormal data.
- Students will demonstrate safe administration of oral medication.
- Students will demonstrate insertion of an indwelling urinary catheter.
- Students will verbalize a comprehensive patient report.

Acute Patient Information

It is the day shift (0700) and students will provide care to William Hampton, a 78-year-old male patient who was admitted to the medical unit two days ago with a primary diagnosis of congestive heart failure (CHF). William presented to his primary physician's clinic with a two day history of weakness, shortness of breath, and difficulty ambulating distances of more than 10 feet. He reports that he has been unable to get out of bed for the past two days. A comparison of William's weight from a previous visit two weeks ago indicated an 11 pound weight increase. William also reports that he rarely needs his PRN oxygen but has used it continuously for the past two days.

William is alert and orientated to person, place, and time. The night nurse reports that his respirations were 38 breaths per minute with ambulation to the bathroom. The nurse counseled him to use a urinal for energy conservation. She has received an order for an indwelling urinary catheter and delegates this task to you. William rested off and on throughout the night, voiding a total of 400 mL. His last set of vital signs at 0530 was: 26 respirations/minute at rest; apical pulse irregular 92 beats/minute; blood pressure 118/70; tympanic temperature 99.5 °F; and oxygen saturation 91% on 2 liters of oxygen per nasal cannula. William denies any pain or discomfort. The 0630 lab results are as follows: B-type natriuretic peptide (BNP) 2300 pg/mL; serum potassium 4.2 mEq/L; and white blood cell count (WBC) 16.2 μ/L. William has a 20 gauge saline lock (SL) in his left forearm. No intravenous (IV) fluids are infusing.

Bilateral course crackles were auscultated by the night nurse. William has a frequent productive cough of clear sputum. His bowel sounds are active and he reports feeling hungry for breakfast. The night nurse reported 2+ pitting edema bilaterally in William's ankles and feet. Pedal pulses were difficult to palpate. As of this morning William's weight is down six pounds since his admission two days ago. William slept with the head of the bed elevated 45 degrees.

William lives alone. He speaks frequently of his late wife who died two years ago; they had been married for 55 years. Many grandchildren take turns visiting him daily. He is now considering getting a pet to help decrease the feeling of being in an empty house. William enjoys talking about current events and frequently watches news channels on TV. The night nurse jokes, "I hope you are up to date on current events" as she leaves for the day. Students will begin care of William at 0730; the educator may set a visible clock for this time.

Other Relevant Patient Information

- Medical diagnoses include: CHF, atrial fibrillation, chronic obstructive pulmonary disease (COPD), hypertension (HTN), and hypothyroidism
- Past history of smoking: began smoking at the age of 14, quit 10 years ago
- Height 6'0"
- Morning weight today was 235 pounds
- Current medications: all medications are via the oral route unless indicated otherwise: multivitamin one daily, Colace 100 mg daily, Synthroid 75 mcg daily, Coreg 25 mg twice a day, Lasix 40 mg twice a day, KDur 20 mEq twice a day, Digoxin 0.25 mg daily, Zestril 10 mg daily, ASA EC 81 mg daily, Zithromax 250 mg daily, Advair 250/50 one puff twice a day, and albuterol nebulizer 1 unit dose every 4–6 hours as needed.
- Allergies: sulfa

Guidelines for Student Preparation

For student success, a review of the following medications and skills are required prior to the simulation exercise. Be sure to review Chapter 1 for further student guidelines. As students review medications the following information should be noted: the trade and generic names, the indications of each medication, safe dosage ranges, primary nursing implications, and common side effects.

- Review pre-steps to patient care: handwashing, introduction of self to the patient, verifying patient identification via two identifiers (name & date of birth), ensuring privacy, and utilization of gloves and personal protective equipment (PPE) when necessary.
- Medications used within this simulation include: multivitamin, Colace, Synthroid, Coreg, Lasix, K-Dur, Digoxin, Zestril, ASA, Zithromax, Advair, and an albuterol nebulizer PRN.
- Students should review dosage calculations prior to the simulation exercise as they will be required during medication administration.
- Students should be familiar with the procedure of flushing a saline lock (SL).
- Students should fully review the data collection process. Be aware that a patient chart will be available for review during the simulation exercise. The data collection nurse should share any abnormal findings with the team leader.
- Students should be able to demonstrate how to manually obtain all patient vital signs including blood pressure, apical pulse, respirations, oxygen saturation, and temperature. Understand the HPS functions to increase competency of these skills.
- Students will be required to calculate the intake and output for the patient within this simulation exercise.

- Students should be familiar with the insertion of an indwelling urinary catheter.
- Students should be prepared to administer an albuterol nebulizer, as it is a PRN medication.
- Students should review the application of oxygen via various methods.
- Students should review the process of giving a verbal report to the RN supervisor.
- Students must demonstrate therapeutic communication with the patient and family member. Speak to the HPS and ask questions. The educator will provide patient responses.
- Students must be able to understand the following lab values: B-type natriuretic peptide (BNP), serum potassium (K+), and white blood cell count (WBC). What data should be collected with these lab values in mind?
- Students may report any concerns which arise during the simulation event to the RN supervisor.
- Students must demonstrate proper documentation of medications on the medication administration record (MAR). Information during the simulation event such as vital signs should be recorded for later use in documentation.

Student Simulation Roles

The student simulation roles are as follows: a team leader, medication nurse, data collection nurse, and family member. The educator may choose to restructure roles as deemed necessary. For further review of the student roles refer to Chapter 1 of this text. Roles may be assigned prior to the simulation exercise start. It is imperative that students are prepared for all potential roles. As this is a team effort, students may consult each other as the simulation exercise progresses. Accuracy needs to be ensured and students may choose to double-check the patient's vital signs and the medications being administered. The educator may reserve the right to grade students on an individual basis, especially if one member of the team is clearly unprepared for the exercise.

Simulation Grade

The educator will provide specific information related to the grading of the simulation exercise. The student's grade will be affected by the timely completion of skills with accuracy. If this is the first simulation exercise students have participated in the grading grid may be followed with the final evaluation resulting in a pass or fail. The grading grid presented within this text recommends the following guidelines for grade construction.

1. **Beginning Steps (10%):** This includes washing your hands, introducing yourself to the patient, explaining the plan of care, checking the proper patient identification (use two indicators), providing privacy, and donning gloves or applying the appropriate PPE as necessary.

2. **Data Collection (30%):** Prioritize the collection of data; recall the ABC's (airway, breathing, and circulation). Data collection should remain focused on key patient priorities. The vital signs will be manual to ensure that students can accurately obtain an apical pulse, respirations, and blood pressure. Students should demonstrate the usage of all needed equipment. For example, to obtain the patient's oxygen saturation, correctly apply the device and wait for the educator to verbally provide the reading. Students should further expand upon the patient information learned in report. Subjective and objective data should be gathered. Data collection should include inspection of the anterior and posterior HPS surfaces. Take care not to damage the HPS while turning it.

3. **Implementation (30%):** Performance of nursing skills needs to be done in an accurate and timely manner. See the above information for content to review. Students will be required to administer some of the medications listed above. Be sure to review all guidelines of medication administration listed in Chapter 1. Dosage calculation must be performed within this simulation. If a question arises during medication administration, inform the team leader, who will address the issue. Significant points may be deducted for medication errors. Students should be prepared to insert an indwelling urinary catheter.

4. **Evaluation (10%):** Evaluate each intervention performed. After students perform an action, question if the action resulted in the desired outcome; if not, the formulation of other interventions may be required. Evaluate the medications administered to determine if the desired effect of the medication occurred. Pre-plan how to evaluate each medication administered. Reassessment of vital signs is required.

5. **Verbal Report (10%):** Upon the conclusion of the simulation exercise students will be required to provide a verbal report to the RN supervisor. The verbal report should be clear, concise, and organized. Effective communication must be demonstrated.

6. **Student Professionalism (10%):** Professional dress, proper communication, display of teamwork, preparedness for the scenario, and

adaptation to stress will make up the final portion of the simulation grade.

Family Member Information

Your grandfather is a very kind man. He lives alone. You are from a large family and he does receive daily visits from family members. The family has discussed aiding him in obtaining a pet as suggested by his family physician. He complained about an increase in weakness and difficulty ambulating a few days ago, so another relative brought him in for an evaluation, after which point he was admitted to the hospital. He does try to follow most of his doctor's recommendations. However, he eats a lot of canned soup and processed foods high in salt. You feel that he does this for ease of meal preparation. Your grandfather is mentally sharp because he "always keeps his mind going with current events." In fact, you would say that you get a great deal of information regarding current events from him.

Case Study for Simulation 1 Data Collection & Medication Administration (Adult)

1. Mr. Hampton asks you to explain to him what CHF means. How would you describe the condition in terms the patient can understand?
2. The nurse recalls that both right- and left-sided heart failure are potential diagnoses for patients. Compare the two in a table.
3. What is the best way to evaluate a patient's fluid volume status? What is your rationale for this answer?
4. Mr. Hampton had the following intake and output amounts during your shift:

    Breakfast—6oz. glass of orange juice, one carton of milk (240 mL), and one cup of coffee (280 mL)

    Lunch—6oz. of cranberry juice and one carton of milk (240 mL)

    You note that he drank an estimated 400 mL from his bedside water pitcher.

    Output—Voided 400 mL at 0845, voided 250 mL at 1030, voided 400 mL at 1230, voided 300 mL at 1400.

    Using the information above to calculate Mr. Hampton's intake and output for your shift.

5. As you auscultate Mr. Hampton's lung sounds, you hear crackles. Describe what crackles indicate and what other important information to consider as a result of this finding.
6. What is the primary action of Synthroid? Explain a rationale for why it is scheduled to be administered at 0630.

Mr. Hampton questions why he is on more than one medication for his high blood pressure. Answer the following questions related to Mr. Hampton's hypertension.

7. Which of the medications in this simulation are indicated to reduce blood pressure? Why might multiple medications be ordered?
8. Is Mr. Hampton's blood pressure effectively controlled? What is your rationale for this answer?
9. In report, you learned that Mr. Hampton's BNP is 2300, his potassium is 4.2, and his WBC is 16.2. Why was this information important for the night nurse to report?
10. Reflection is a vital part of the learning process. Discuss what went well during the simulation experience and what areas need improvement.
11. Chart on the care that you provided Mr. Hampton per the educator's guidelines.

2

Urinary & Pyelonephritis (Adult)

Goals/Outcomes of Simulation Exercise

- Students will demonstrate data collection related to the urinary system.
- Students will demonstrate skills of obtaining a urine specimen and medication administration.
- Students will educate the patient on plan of care for urinary tract infection and safe sexual practices.

Acute Patient Information

It is the evening shift (1500) and students will provide care to Nanna Krause, a 21-year-old female patient who was admitted with a primary diagnosis of pyelonephritis. Nanna reports that she began having signs and symptoms of a urinary tract infection five days ago. Nanna states she experienced a burning sensation with urination, had mild abdominal pain, and had frequent urgent urination. She states, "I seriously had to go every 10 minutes." Nanna was advised by her good friend to take cranberry capsules, vitamin C tablets, and phenazopyridine. She began taking the medications after she researched them on the Internet because "they seemed to be what I needed." Nanna awoke this morning with a high fever, vomiting, and severe abdominal pain. Nanna further adds that she had moderate bilateral flank pain.

Nanna reports that she began having frequent urinary tract infections about the time she began college. She stated, "I know what they feel like." She vomited in the emergency department at 1300. Nanna has a 20 gauge IV in her left hand with a 0.9% sodium chloride (NaCl) 1,000 mL bolus infusing at 250 mL/hr. She has refused any oral intake. She voided 50 mL of cloudy, foul smelling, dark amber urine in the emergency department. Her last set of vital signs at 1400 were: respirations 14 per minute at rest; regular apical pulse 90 beats per minute; blood pressure 124/70; tympanic temperature 104.3 °F, and oxygen saturation 98% on room air.

The admitting lab results were as follows: pregnancy text negative; white blood cell count (WBC) 22.0 µL, blood urea nitrogen (BUN) 24 mg/dL, and gonorrhea and chlamydia cultures are pending. Nanna's urinalysis results were as follows: + red blood cells, + white blood cells, and + nitrites. The physician has ordered a mini catheterization to be done to obtain a sample for the urine culture. Medication orders have been sent to the pharmacy, and the IV antibiotics should be started after the mini catheterization.

Nanna's lung sounds are clear and her heart tones are regular. Bowel sounds are present. Her last bowel movement was yesterday and was reported to be "normal." Her abdomen is soft and tender to palpation. Pedal pulses are present and strong. Morphine 4 mg IV was administered in the emergency department (ED) an hour ago. She last rated her pain at 2 of 5 stating, "The morphine really helped."

Other Relevant Patient Information

- Past medical diagnoses: three urinary tract infections in the past year
- Past history of smoking: began two years ago, smokes a few cigarettes on the weekends "when she goes out"
- Alcohol intake: five to six beers on Friday and Saturday nights
- Frequent sexual activity with no use of birth control
- Height 5' 5"

- Weight 125 pounds
- Current medications: cranberry capsules two twice a day, vitamin C tablets one tablet twice a day, and phenazopyridine. She states, "I can't remember if that one was once or twice a day" in reference to the phenazopyridine. The patient is uncertain of any of the medication dosages; no routine medications
- Allergies: none

Guidelines for Student Preparation

For student success, a review of the following medications and skills are required prior to the simulation exercise. Be sure to review Chapter 1 for further student guidelines. As students review medications the following information should be noted: the trade and generic names, the indications of each medication, safe dosage ranges, primary nursing implications, and common side effects.

- Medications used within this simulation include: Vicodin, ciprofloxacin (IV), Zofran oral disintegrating tablets (ODT), and 0.9% sodium chloride (NaCl).
- Students will be required to administer a secondary IV medication (ciprofloxacin).
- Students should be familiar with specific considerations of narcotic administration.
- Students should fully review the data collection process. Review the provided patient chart during the simulation exercise.
- Student will be required to demonstrate how to obtain a full set of vital signs.
- Students will be required to demonstrate a mini catheterization.
- Students must verbalize therapeutic communication with the HPS. Review the patient information above. Pre-plan how you provide education on the topics identified in the patient history and per the friend.
- Students should review the process of giving a verbal report upon the conclusion of the simulation exercise to the RN supervisor.
- Students must demonstrate proper documentation of medications on the medication administration record (MAR). In addition, information during the simulation event, such as vital signs, should be recorded by students for later documentation.

Student Simulation Roles

The student simulation roles are as follows: team leader, medication nurse, data collection nurse, and friend. The educator may choose to restructure roles as deemed necessary. For further review of the student roles refer to Chapter 1 of the student text. Roles may be assigned prior to the simulation exercise start. It is imperative that students are prepared for all potential roles. Students may consult each other as the simulation exercise progresses. Accuracy needs to be ensured and students may choose to double-check the patient's vital signs and the medications being administered. The educator may reserve the right to grade students on an individual basis, especially if one member of the team is clearly unprepared for the exercise.

Simulation Grade

The educator will provide specific information related to the grading of the simulation exercise. The student's grade will be affected by the timely completion of skills with accuracy. The grading grid presented within this text recommends the following guidelines for grade construction.

1. Beginning Steps (10%): This includes washing hands, introducing oneself to the patient, explaining the plan of care, checking the proper patient identification (use two indicators), providing privacy, and donning gloves or applying the appropriate personal protective equipment (PPE) as necessary.

2. Data Collection (30%): Prioritize data collection. Data collection should remain focused on key patient priorities. Vital signs will be manual to ensure that students can accurately obtain an apical pulse and respirations. Students should demonstrate the usage of all needed equipment. For example, to obtain the patient's oxygen saturation, correctly apply the device and wait for the educator to verbally provide the reading. Subjective and objective data should be gathered. Be sure to obtain data related to the patient's psychosocial history.

3. Implementation (30%): Performance of various nursing skills needs to be done in an accurate and timely manner. See the above information for content to review. Significant points may be deducted if a medication error is made. Students will be required to perform a mini catheterization and administer an IV antibiotic. It is expected that students provide the patient education related to: (a) urinary tract infection prevention and (b) safe sexual practices. Students should pre-plan information for patient education.

4. Evaluation (10%): Evaluate each intervention performed. After students perform an action they should question if the action resulted in the desired outcome. Evaluation for this simulation may include repeated vital signs, reviewing pain status, and evaluation of patient education.

5. Verbal Report (10%): Upon the conclusion of the simulation exercise students will be required to provide a verbal report to the RN supervisor. The verbal report should be clear, concise, and organized. Effective communication must be demonstrated.

6. Student Professionalism (10%): Professional dress, proper communication, display of teamwork, preparedness for the scenario, and adaptation to stress will make up the final portion of the simulation grade.

Family Member Information (Friend)

You brought Nanna to the emergency room. The two of you have been friends since high school. Though you consider Nanna a great friend you are really worried about the choices she has begun to make now that she is away from home. She parties all night Friday and Saturday. She typically drinks heavy amounts of alcohol on the weekends. She used to be a star athlete in high school, especially in track and field. She has begun to smoke, which is something that she was opposed to in high school. Nanna has begun to have "adult relationships" with multiple men, of which you do not approve. You pull a nurse aside and ask her to speak to Nanna about the risk of pregnancy and sexually transmitted diseases. Nanna might listen to a professional about this topic. You have tried to discuss this topic with her in the past but are "just too embarrassed."

Case Study for Simulation 2
Urinary & Pyelonephritis (Adult)

1. Nanna reports taking cranberry capsules, vitamin C tablets, and phenazopyridine. Why might these medications be helpful to patients who have a urinary tract infection (UTI)?
2. What are the risk factors for urinary tract infections?
3. List the signs and symptoms of pyelonephritis.
4. Nanna's increased sexual activity correlates with frequent UTIs. Why might sexual activity increase Nanna's risk of a UTI? How can this risk be reduced?
5. To assist Nanna in the prevention of UTIs, what information should be reviewed?
6. Reflection is a vital part of the learning process. Discuss what went well during the simulation experience and what areas need improvement.
7. Chart on the care that you provided Nanna per the educator's guidelines.

Orthopedic Surgery & Deep Vein Thrombosis (Adult)

Goals/Outcomes of Simulation Exercise

- Students will collect data on a postoperative patient and recognize abnormal findings.
- Students will report abnormal findings from data collection to supervisor.
- Students will demonstrate skills of oral and subcutaneous medication administration.
- Students will evaluate effectiveness of nursing interventions.

Acute Patient Information

It is the day shift (0700) and students will provide care to Patrick Handlon, a 53-year-old male who had a left total knee replacement three days ago. Today he will be discharged home. He has a history of osteoarthritis in both knees. Postoperative progress has been considered normal up to this point. Physical and occupational therapy have conducted a discharge evaluation and he is ready to be discharged home. Patrick uses a continuous passive motion (CPM) machine three to four times a day. His pain is controlled with two hydrocodone/acetaminophen tablets every four to six hours. Estimated blood loss during surgery was 400 mL. Patrick's hemoglobin today was 9.2 g/dL (stated in labs later in the scenario). Significant ecchymosis is reported in the entire left leg from the thigh to ankle. He has an anti-embolism stocking on the right leg. A dressing has been applied over the left knee incision and an ACE (elastic) wrap covers the dressing down to his mid-calf region.

Patrick is irritable and anxious to go home. He was restless throughout the night shift. Hydroxyzine was administered in addition to the hydrocodone/acetaminophen to keep pain at a "1–2" on a scale of 0–5 for the night nurse. At 0600 vital signs were as follows: blood pressure 172/98; apical pulse 72 beats per minute; respirations 22 per minute; tympanic temperature 99.8 °F; and oxygen saturation 94% on room air. The 0600 lab results were as follows: white blood cell count (WBC) 11 μL, hemoglobin (Hgb) 9.2 g/dL, and hematocrit (Hct) 25%. He has an 18 gauge saline lock in the right hand.

Patrick's lung sounds are diminished but clear. He had a large bowel movement early this morning. He complains of a poor appetite. He needs to be reminded to use his incentive spirometer, tells the nurses he is not interested in it, and states, "Quit bothering me about it." He refused to ambulate to the bathroom during the night and used a urinal. Equal bilateral pedal pulses are palpated. Edema is observed in the left lower leg and is rated at a 3 +.

Patrick has been awake on and off all night and became more restless toward morning. He states that he seems to be having "a lot of pain in my left calf." The night nurse reports he was last medicated for pain at 0300. Students will begin care of Patrick at 0730.

Other Relevant Patient Information

- Height 5'11"
- Weight 210 pounds
- Previous medical diagnoses include: hypertension, gastric reflux
- Current medications: hydrochlorothiazide (HCTZ) 25 mg daily, Protonix 40 mg daily, hydrocodone/acetaminophen 7.5/500 mg 1–2 tablets

every 4 hours PRN knee pain, hydroxyzine 25 mg every 4 hours PRN knee pain, Colace 100 mg twice daily, multivitamin daily, and Coumadin 5 mg daily
- Allergies: penicillin (PCN)

Guidelines for Student Preparation

For student success, a review of the following medications and skills are required prior to the simulation exercise. Be sure to review Chapter 1 for further student guidelines. As students review medications the following information should be noted: the trade and generic names, the indications of each medication, safe dosage ranges, primary nursing implications, and common side effects.

- Medications used within this simulation include: hydrochlorothiazide (HCTZ), Protonix, multivitamin, hydrocodone/acetaminophen, hydroxyzine, coumadin and Heparin (subcutaneous).
- Students should fully review the data collection process. Be aware that a patient chart will be available for review during the simulation exercise.
- Students should be able to demonstrate how to manually obtain all patient vital signs including blood pressure, apical pulse, respirations, oxygen saturation, and temperature.
- Students should review the application of oxygen via various methods.
- Students must demonstrate proper data collection technique related to patient pain.
- Students should be able to evaluate changes in patient condition within the scenario.
- Students should review the process associated with providing a comprehensive verbal report to a RN supervisor.
- Students must verbalize therapeutic communication.
- Students must be able to understand the following lab values: white blood cell count (WBC), hemoglobin (Hgb), hematocrit (Hct), partial thromboplastin time (PTT), and pro-time (PT).
- Students must demonstrate proper documentation of medications on the medication administration record (MAR). Students may be required to write a nursing note in relation to the simulation events.

Student Simulation Roles

The student simulation roles are as follows: a team leader, medication nurse, data collection nurse, and family member. The educator may choose to restructure roles as deemed necessary. For further review of the student roles refer to Chapter 1 of this text. Roles may be assigned prior to the simulation exercise start. It is imperative that students are prepared for all potential roles. Students may consult each other as the simulation exercise progresses. Accuracy needs to be ensured and students may choose to double-check the patient's vital signs and the medications being administered. The educator may reserve the right to grade students on an individual basis, especially if one member of the group is clearly unprepared for the exercise.

Simulation Grade

The educator will provide specific information related to the grading of the simulation exercise. The student's grade will be affected by the timely completion of skills with accuracy. The grading grid presented within this text recommends the following guidelines for grade construction.

1. Beginning Steps: (10%): This includes washing your hands, introducing yourself to the patient, explaining the plan of care, checking the proper patient identification (use two indicators), providing privacy, and donning gloves or applying the appropriate PPE as necessary.

2. Data Collection (30%): Prioritize data collection; recall the ABC's (airway, breathing, and circulation). Data collection should remain focused on key patient priorities. The first set of vital signs will be manual to ensure that students can accurately obtain an apical pulse, respirations, and blood pressure. Students should demonstrate the usage of all needed equipment. For example, to obtain the patient's oxygen saturation correctly, apply the device and wait for the educator to verbally provide the reading.

3. Report (10%): Students will need to notify the RN supervisor of the change in patient condition. Written physician's orders obtained by the supervisor will be delegated to the PN students.

4. Implementation (30%): Performance of various nursing skills needs to be done in an accurate and timely manner. See the above information for content to review. Orders will be given for the team to carry out. Be sure to implement the physician's orders in a timely fashion. Students should communicate with other departments (i.e. lab, EKG, and x-ray) the orders which need to be carried out.

5. Evaluation (10%): Evaluate each intervention performed. After students perform an action they should question if the action resulted in the desired outcome; if not, the formulation of other interventions may be required. Evaluate all medications administered. Re-check the patient's vital signs and pain level, as this is required.

6. Student Professionalism (10%): Professional dress, proper communication, display of teamwork, preparedness for the scenario, and adaptation to stress will make up the final portion of the simulation grade.

Family Member Information

Patrick is used to being active but has had increased knee pain over the past six months. He is a teacher at an elementary school and hopes that this surgery will help with his activity level. He is married and has three grown children and three grandchildren. As the family member you are concerned that he will do more than he is supposed to do at home. He is stubborn and at times non-compliant when it comes to his heath care. When you came in today to take him home he seemed to be much more agitated. You wonder what may have occurred. You are worried about the pain in his left calf and are concerned how you will help care for him at home.

Case Study for Simulation 3 Orthopedic Surgery & Deep Vein Thrombosis (DVT)

1. Patrick has a possible deep vein thrombosis. What are his significant risk factors for a DVT?
2. What are the classic signs and symptoms of a DVT?
3. List priority nursing interventions for Patrick.
4. Discuss interventions to prevent DVTs in hospitalized patients.
5. Reflection is a vital part of the learning process. Discuss what went well during the simulation experience and what areas need improvement.
6. Chart on the care that you provided Patrick per the educator's guidelines.

Cardiac & Acute Coronary Syndrome (Adult)

Goals/Outcomes of Simulation Exercise

- Students will collect data, recognize abnormal findings, and report to the supervisor.
- Students will implement nursing interventions as directed by the RN supervisor.
- Students will evaluate effectiveness of interventions performed.

Acute Patient Information

It is the day shift (0700) and students will provide care to David Arens, a 65-year-old male who sustained a left mid-shaft femoral fracture yesterday when he fell an estimated 15–20 feet from the roof of his barn. David's admitting hemoglobin was 9.0 g/dL. The fractured femur was stabilized during surgery with screws and a plate. Estimated blood loss during surgery was 300 mL. One unit of packed red blood cells (PRBCs) was transfused in the operating room. Significant ecchymosis is reported in the left thigh. No other significant injuries were sustained during the fall.

David is alert and oriented to person, place, and time. He rested well throughout the night shift and his leg pain has been controlled with the use of a morphine patient-controlled analgesia (PCA). He rated his leg pain at a "1–2" on a scale of 0–5 for the night nurse. At 0600 vital signs were as follows: blood pressure 138/86, apical pulse 84 beats per minute, respirations 18 per minute, tympanic temperature 98.8 °F, and oxygen saturation 96% on room air. The 0600 lab results are as follows: white blood cell count (WBC) 12 μL, hemoglobin (Hgb) 9.2 g/dL, and hematocrit (Hct) 26.1%. His indwelling urinary catheter had 850 mL of clear yellow urine output during the night shift. He has an 18 gauge IV in his right forearm infusing 5% dextrose with 0.45% sodium chloride (NaCl) and 20 mEq of potassium chloride (KCl)/liter infusing at 100 mL/hr.

David's lung sounds are clear. He is compliant with his incentive spirometer, using it every hour for five breaths while awake and demonstrating proper usage. He reports mild nausea. David's oral intake during the night consisted of a few ice chips. David's bowel sounds are hypoactive with positive reports of flatus. Equal bilateral pedal pulses are palpated. Slight edema is observed in the left lower leg rated at a 1 +.

David has been awake since 0500. He states that as a farmer he is "used to getting up early." He expresses concerns that he is "stressed" over who will continue to keep his farm up and running while he is in the hospital. He has 60 dairy cows that need to be milked every morning and evening. David informed the night nurse that he does not like to "lay around" and that he rarely watches "the junk on TV." He notes that he may have a hard time with the recovery process. He further stated, "All there is to do is sit and worry about all the things I should be doing." David requested a cigarette multiple times on the night shift. Students will begin care of David at 0730.

Other Relevant Patient Information

- 1/2 pack per day (PPD) smoker since age 25
- Height 5'11"

- Weight 289 pounds
- Previous medical diagnoses include: hypertension, hyperlipidemia, nicotine addiction, and obesity
- David's younger brother Greg had a myocardial infarction (MI) three months ago and underwent a triple bypass; he reports that his dad "died of heart trouble;" his mother is living and is in good health; he has no siblings other than Greg
- Current medications: lisinopril 20 mg daily, hydrochlorothiazide (HCTZ) 50 mg daily, and Zocor 40 mg every evening
- No known allergies

Guidelines for Student Preparation

For student success, a review of the following medications and skills are required prior to the simulation exercise. Be sure to review Chapter 1 for further student guidelines. As students review medications the following information should be noted: the trade and generic names, the indications of each medication, safe dosage ranges, primary nursing implications, and common side effects.

- Medications used within this simulation include: lisinopril, hydrochlorothiazide (HCTZ), Zocor, Lovenox, Claforan, aspirin, morphine (IV), and nitroglycerin (sublingual).
- Students should fully review the data collection process. Be aware that a patient chart will be available for review during the simulation exercise.
- Students should be able to demonstrate how to manually obtain all patient vital signs including blood pressure, apical pulse, respirations, oxygen saturation, and temperature.
- Students should review the application of oxygen via various methods.
- Students must demonstrate data collection related to the patient's pain and the utilization of a patient-controlled analgesia (PCA).
- Students must demonstrate the proper application of a 5-lead cardiac telemetry monitor.
- Students should review the process associated with providing a comprehensive verbal report to an RN supervisor. Once the data collection process is complete, students should report all abnormal findings in a timely manner.
- Students must verbalize therapeutic communication.
- Students must be able to understand the following lab values: white blood cell count (WBC), hemoglobin (Hgb), and hematocrit (Hct).
- Students must demonstrate proper documentation of medications on the medication administration record (MAR). Information during the simulation event, such as vital signs, should be recorded by students for later documentation.

Student Simulation Roles

The student simulation roles are as follows: a team leader, medication nurse, data collection nurse, and family member. The educator may choose to restructure roles as deemed necessary. For further review of the student roles, refer to Chapter 1 of this text. Roles may be assigned just prior to the simulation exercise start. It is imperative that students are prepared for all potential roles. Students may consult each other as the simulation exercise progresses. Students may choose to double-check the patient's vital signs and the medications being administered. The educator may reserve the right to grade students on an individual basis, especially if one member of the group is clearly unprepared for the exercise.

Simulation Grade

The educator will provide specific information related to the grading of the simulation exercise. The student's grade will be affected by the timely completion of skills with accuracy. The grading grid presented within this text recommends the following guidelines for grade construction.

1. Beginning Steps: (10%): This includes washing your hands, introducing yourself to the patient, explaining the plan of care, checking the proper patient identification (use two indicators), providing privacy, and donning gloves or applying the appropriate PPE as necessary.
2. Data Collection (30%): Prioritize the collection of data; recall the ABC's (airway, breathing, and circulation). Data collection should remain focused on key patient priorities. The first set of vital signs will be manual to ensure that students can accurately obtain an apical pulse, respirations, and blood pressure. Students should demonstrate the usage of all needed equipment. For example, to obtain the patient's oxygen saturation, correctly apply the device and wait for the educator to verbally provide the reading. The data collection for this simulation scenario will focus on the cardiac system.
3. Report (10%): Upon the conclusion of data collection, students will need to notify the RN supervisor of changes in the patient's condition and abnormal findings. Students should include important data assessed and collected during verbal report. Clearly communicate all patient concerns. New orders will be delegated after report.
4. Implementation (30%): Performance of various nursing skills needs to be done in an accurate and timely manner. See the above

information for content to review. Medications will be administered via the oral, sublingual, and IV routes. The lab and x-ray departments will need to be notified of new physician's orders.

5. **Evaluation (10%):** Evaluate each intervention performed. After students perform an action question if the action, resulted in the desired outcome. Evaluation for this simulation may include repeated vital signs, reflection on how the HPS responded to medications, and pain status.

6. **Student Professionalism (10%):** Professional dress, proper communication, display of teamwork, preparedness for the scenario, and adaptation to stress will make up the final portion of the simulation grade.

Family Member Information

David was repairing a hail-damaged barn roof when he fell an estimated 15–20 feet. He had been working long hours and was exhausted. David has not been taking good care of himself. He is a "meat and potatoes kind of guy who puts gravy on everything." His primary doctor has encouraged weight loss to reduce his high blood pressure and cholesterol. His younger brother Greg had a triple bypass three months ago. David smokes half a pack of cigarettes per day. He has frequently been asking to go outside to have a cigarette because he claims it will make him feel better. David is a "tough guy" and usually does not complain of pain. The student assigned the role of family member should reassure David that matters relating to his farm are being taken care of. As his condition deteriorates, the student who plays the role of family member should be sure to ask questions about the nursing interventions performed.

Case Study for Simulation 4
Cardiac & Acute Coronary Syndrome

1. David realizes that he might be having a heart attack. He asks you what a heart attack is and how it occurs. You explain that:

2. What are common signs and symptoms of acute coronary syndrome?

3. How frequently will you monitor David's vital signs? What is your rationale for this time frame?

4. A variety of lab tests were ordered on David. Explain why each lab test was ordered.

5. List medical procedures that may be used to treat an acute MI.

6. Lovenox is ordered for this patient postoperative to prevent the formation of a deep vein thrombosis. Should this medication be administered to a patient experiencing chest pain? Why?

7. Reflection is a vital part of the learning process. Discuss what went well during the simulation experience and what areas need improvement.

8. Chart on the care that you provided David per the educator's guidelines.

5

Integument & Wound Care (Adult)

Goals/Outcomes of Simulation Exercise

- Students will demonstrate thorough data collection and report abnormal findings to the supervisor.

- Students will demonstrate use of personal protective equipment (PPE) and application of contact precautions.

- Students will demonstrate skill components of a dressing change and safe medication administration.

- Students will demonstrate therapeutic communication.

Acute Patient Information

It is the day shift (0700) and students will provide care to Shirley Griggs, a 66-year-old female patient who underwent a bowel resection three days ago. A biopsy obtained during a routine colonoscopy tested positive for carcinoma, and a bowel resection was recommended. During surgery a segment of the large bowel and several lymph nodes were removed. A small abscess was discovered and the surgical wound was left open. The exact cause of the abscess could not be determined, but the surgeon believes it may have formed as a complication of a ruptured diverticulum. A culture was obtained and Shirley tested positive for methicillin-resistant staphylococcus aureus (MRSA); results posted this morning. No fecal diversion (colostomy) was created during the surgery.

Shirley has an open midline abdominal incision that measures 9 cm in length by 3 cm in width by 2 cm in depth. Personal protective equipment (PPE) must be utilized and contact precautions have been instituted. The supervisor informs you that he will notify the physician on morning rounds of the MRSA-positive culture. He states, "New orders for an antibiotic may be given later this morning." During the last dressing change the nurse reported the following information: (a) moderate amount of yellow-brown exudate, (b) the wound base was beefy red with granulation, and (c) a slight foul odor. Shirley tolerated the last dressing change without difficulty. Today is Shirley's postoperative day number three. Shirley is alert and orientated to person, place, and time. The night nurse reports that she rested well and has been using her morphine patient-controlled analgesia (PCA) as needed; 8 mg was self-administered throughout the night (2300–0630). Shirley reported slight nausea during the night shift.

Shirley's last set of vital signs at 0600 were as follows: respirations 16 per minute at rest; regular apical pulse 76 beats per minute at rest; blood pressure 134/78; tympanic temperature 100.2 °F; and oxygen saturation 97% on room air. The 0600 lab results are as follows: white blood cell count (WBC) 17.4 µL, hemoglobin (Hgb) 10.2 g/dL, and albumin 2.5 g/dL. Shirley has a 20 gauge IV in her left forearm infusing dextrose 5% with 0.45% of sodium chloride (NaCl) with 20 mEq of potassium chloride (KCl)/liter at 75 mL/hr. She is currently receiving a full liquid diet.

The night nurse reports that Shirley's lung sounds were clear but diminished in the bases. She has an occasional cough with minimal sputum production. Bowel sounds are hypoactive. Shirley reports flatus. The night nurse reported slight pedal edema. Pedal pulses were present and strong. She voided 250 mL of clear urine with no difficulty at 0530.

The night nurse states that Shirley is very concerned about her diagnosis of cancer and "what the future holds." She becomes teary eyed when she discusses the diagnosis stating, "I know they caught it early, but it still really scares me." Shirley has also commented on the fact that she feels so "contaminated" with everyone in gowns and gloves. She states, "I want to see my grandkids." Shirley further relays that she comes from a large family and visiting with them is important. She does not want to "spread germs." An oncologist will make rounds later this morning to further review prognosis and further treatment recommendations.

Other Relevant Patient Information

- Past medical diagnoses: osteoporosis, hypertension, and diverticulitis
- Previous surgeries: hysterectomy at age 54
- Past history of smoking: began smoking at the age of 16, 1 pack per day, quit at age 54 following hysterectomy surgery
- Height 5'3"
- Weight 140 pounds
- Current medications: Multivitamin one tablet daily, calcium 600 mg plus vitamin D 200 IU one tablet daily, Hyzaar 50/12.5 mg daily in the morning, and ASA EC 81 mg daily in the morning; all medications listed are via the oral route
- Allergies: no known food or drug allergies

Guidelines for Student Preparation

For student success, a review of the following medications and skills are required prior to the simulation exercise. Be sure to review Chapter 1 for further student guidelines. As students review medications the following information should be noted: the trade and generic names, the indications of each medication, safe dosage ranges, primary nursing implications, and common side effects.

- Medications used within this simulation include: Claforan intravenous (IV), morphine PCA, multivitamin, calcium + vitamin D, Hyzaar, and ASA. Primary IV fluid of 5% dextrose with 0.45% of NaCl and 20 mEq of KCl/liter will be infusing. Ensure that the fluid is infusing at the ordered rate.
- Students should review how to calculate IV fluid infusion rates.
- A morphine PCA is ordered. Review the nursing implications related to this method of medication delivery.
- Students should fully review the data collection process. Be aware that a patient chart will be available for review during the simulation exercise.
- Review data relating to instituting contact precautions in a patient with MRSA. Understand how to correctly apply and remove personal protective equipment (PPE).
- Students will be required to demonstrate how to obtain a full set of vital signs on the human patient simulator (HPS).
- Educate the patient on proper usage of incentive spirometry.

- Students must demonstrate how to perform a dressing change. Measurement and data collection of the wound will be required. Pre-medication prior to the dressing change is required. Review proper terms/vocabulary which should be used to describe a wound.
- Students must demonstrate therapeutic communication. Review the patient information above; pre-plan how you will comfort the patient.
- Fully review the information provided to the family member. Pre-plan how to answer and address the family member's questions and concerns.
- Students should be able to understand how the following lab values affect wound healing: white blood cell count (WBC), hemoglobin (Hgb), and albumin.
- Students should review the process of giving an oral report to the RN supervisor upon the conclusion of the simulation exercise.
- Students must demonstrate proper documentation of medications on the medication administration record (MAR). Information during the simulation event, such as vital signs, should be recorded by students for later documentation.

Student Simulation Roles

The student simulation roles are as follows: a team leader, medication nurse, data collection nurse, and family member (son/daughter). The educator may choose to restructure roles as deemed necessary. For further review of the student roles refer to Chapter 1. Roles may be assigned just prior to the simulation exercise start. It is imperative that students are prepared for all potential roles. Students may consult each other as the simulation exercise progresses. Students may choose to double-check the patient's vital signs and the medications being administered. The educator may reserve the right to grade students on an individual basis, especially if one member of the team is clearly unprepared for the exercise.

Simulation Grade

The educator will provide specific information related to the grading of the simulation exercise. The student's grade will be affected by the timely completion of skills with accuracy. The grading grid presented within this text recommends the following guidelines for grade construction.

1. Beginning Steps (10%): This includes washing hands, introducing yourself to the patient, explaining the plan of care, checking the proper patient identification (use two indicators), providing

privacy, and donning gloves or applying the appropriate personal protective equipment (PPE) as necessary. Carefully review the PPE guidelines for contact precautions. Understand how to correctly apply PPE and what items should be donned.

2. Data Collection (30%): Prioritize the collection of data; recall the ABC's (airway, breathing, and circulation). Data collection should remain focused on key patient priorities. Vital signs will be manual to ensure that students can accurately obtain an apical pulse, blood pressure, and respirations. Students should demonstrate the usage of all needed equipment. For example, to obtain the patient's oxygen saturation, correctly apply the device and wait for the educator to verbally provide the reading. Wound care is a priority for this simulation exercise. Understand how to measure and collect data on wound status. Use proper terms and vocabulary when assessing the wound.

3. Implementation (30%): Performance of various nursing skills needs to be done in an accurate and timely manner. See the above information of content to review. Medications will be administered, including a secondary IV antibiotic. Significant points may be deducted for medication errors. A dressing change will need to be performed on the patient. Students should review dressing change technique as taught in laboratory or clinical. Pre-medicate the patient prior to the dressing change to reduce pain. Provide holistic care and comfort to the patient through therapeutic communication.

4. Evaluation (10%): Evaluate each intervention performed. After students perform an intervention they should question if the action resulted in the desired outcome. Evaluation for this simulation may include repeated vital signs, reflection on how the patient tolerated the dressing change, pain, and response to emotional support.

5. Verbal Report (10%): Upon the conclusion of the simulation exercise students will be required to provide a verbal report to the nurse who will continue patient care. The verbal report should be clear, concise, and organized. Effective communication must be demonstrated.

6. Student Professionalism (10%): Professional dress, proper communication, display of teamwork, preparedness for the scenario, and adaptation to stress will make up the final portion of the simulation grade.

Family Member Information

You arrive to visit your mother today and question the need for gowns and gloves. Is this all really necessary? Do I have to wear a gown and gloves too? I have two small children at home. The discharge nurse spoke with you about changing your mother's dressing daily when she goes home. The physician would like dressing changes done daily, and the patient requests a family member do the procedure. You specifically came today to observe the dressing change. You are feeling optimistic today because the surgeon reported the cancer had not spread to any other areas. You are thankful she had the routine colonoscopy.

Case Study for Simulation 5
Integument & Wound Care (Adult)

1. Shirley's colorectal cancer was discovered during a routine colonoscopy. Discuss the recommendations for when a colonoscopy should be performed. What are the associated risk factors of colorectal cancer?

2. A morphine PCA is ordered. Discuss the nursing considerations of a morphine PCA. What side effects should the nurse monitor for?

3. The following lab results were reported: white blood cell count (WBC) 17.4 µL, hemoglobin (Hgb) 10.2 g/dL, and serum albumin 2.5 g/dL. Discuss how these lab results relate to wound healing.

4. Shirley is diagnosed with methicillin-resistant staphylococcus aureus (MRSA) in her surgical wound. Discuss the contact precautions that must be followed by hospital staff. What medications are primarily used to treat MRSA?

5. Granulation tissue was observed during the last dressing change. Describe the appearance of granulation tissue and why it is important to note.

6. Shirley is currently receiving a full liquid diet. Is a full liquid diet the best choice for this patient? Why or why not?

7. Diminished lung sounds were reported by the night nurse. Discuss the cause of diminished lung sounds, complications that may arise, and ways to improve lung sounds.

8. In addition to a patient's physical needs, nurses must also address emotional components of patient care. List the data obtained within the simulation that describes Shirley's emotional wellbeing. What interventions might the nurse implement related to Shirley's current emotional state?

9. Reflection is a vital part of the learning process. Discuss what went well during the simulation experience and what areas need improvement.

10. Chart on the care that you provided Shirley Griggs per the educator's guidelines.

Cancer & End of Life (Adult)

Goals/Outcomes of Simulation Exercise

- Students will demonstrate data collection and identify abnormal data.

- Students will prioritize nursing care for the patient with end of life issues.

- Students will apply principles of asepsis for the neutropenic patient's protection.

- Students will verbalize effective communication to members of the health care team.

Acute Patient Information

It is the evening shift (1500) and students will provide care to Jean Hafner, a 55-year-old female patient with stage IV pancreatic cancer. She was a pack-a-day smoker for over 35 years and quit smoking when cancer was discovered 5 months ago. Jean underwent a laparoscopic Whipple procedure. She had a slow recovery from the surgery and a jejunostomy tube was inserted for feedings. Treatments of chemotherapy with gemcitabine were given after her recovery from Whipple surgery. Jean has an implanted port in her left upper chest for chemotherapy. She has been receiving parenteral nutrition at night due to improper functioning of her jejunostomy tube. She is hospitalized to have the jejunostomy tube removed and for pain control. On admission she had severe abdominal pain, a fever, and a history of low neutrophil count three days ago. Current lab reports are pending. Reverse isolation precautions have been instituted.

Jean is quiet and is confused at times. She knows who she is but has no idea why she is hospitalized or what the year is. She was admitted directly from her home after the home care nurse saw her this morning and phoned her oncologist for admitting orders. She is just getting settled in her room now by the certified nursing assistant while you are getting a report from the admitting RN. He reports that Jean is alert but has periods of confusion. Her skin is hot to touch and she is too weak to ambulate. Jean voided a small amount of dark amber urine on admission. Her vitals were as follows: blood pressure 92/58, apical pulse 48 beats per minute, respirations 22 breaths per minute, tympanic temperature 101.4 °F, and oxygen saturation 83% on room air. She has an implanted port in the left chest that has been accessed. Lactated ringers (LR) is infusing at a rate of 85 mL/hr. She has decreased breath sounds bilaterally. Her abdomen is slightly distended with no bowel sounds. The admitting nurse has inserted a nasogastric tube (NG) per physician's orders. Jean rates her pain at a 5 of 5. She states, "The pain is mostly in my stomach but I hurt all over." The admitting nurse also tells you that Jean is talking about dying and her wish is to die at home.

There are no lab results for Jean at this time but you are told by family that her white counts "were very low three days ago." Clinic records confirm the low WBC count. Labs were drawn from the implanted port when accessed and are pending. Jean has a fentanyl duragesic patch 25 mcg/hr applied.

The admission nurse states that Jean came in with one family member who is very concerned about her. He says the family member seems to understand how sick Jean is. Jean lives alone 30 miles from town. Various family members feel 30 miles is too far for them to continue driving daily to care for her at home. Plans for Jean to be admitted to the hospice unit in town are in progress. Jean does not want to leave her home and repeatedly tells the family she wishes to die at home. Family members have been arguing in the process of making end of life decisions.

Other Relevant Patient Information

- Past medical diagnoses: pancreatic cancer stage IV, diabetes mellitus type II, and hypertension
- Previous surgeries: laparoscopic Whipple 5 months ago, bilateral total hip prosthesis due to osteoarthritis, hysterectomy at age 45
- Past history of smoking; began smoking at the age of 20, 1 pack per day, quit when diagnosed with pancreatic cancer
- Height 5'5"
- Weight 100 pounds
- Current medications: fentanyl duragesic patch 25 mcg/hr, Zofran oral disintegrating tablets (ODT) 4 mg as needed for nausea, parenteral nutrition at night including lipids
- Allergies: penicillin and codeine

Guidelines for Student Preparation

For student success, a review of the following medications and skills are required prior to the simulation exercise. Be sure to review Chapter 1 for further student guidelines. As students review medications the following information should be noted: the trade and generic names, the indications of each medication safe dosage ranges, primary nursing implications, and common side effects.

- Medications used within this simulation include: Fentanyl duragesic patch 25 mcg/hr, Zofran oral disintegrating tablets (ODT), and lactated ringers (LR) IV.
- Students should fully review the data collection process. Be aware that a patient chart will be available for review during the simulation exercise.
- Students should be able to demonstrate how to manually obtain all patient vital signs including blood pressure, apical pulse, respirations, oxygen saturation, and temperature.
- Students should review the application of oxygen via various methods.
- Students must demonstrate proper data collection techniques related to the patient's pain and end of life cares.
- Students must verbalize therapeutic communication.

Student Simulation Roles

The student simulation roles are as follows: a team leader, medication nurse, data collection nurse, and family member. The educator may choose to restructure roles as deemed necessary. For further review of the student roles refer to Chapter 1 of this text. Roles may be assigned prior to the simulation exercise start. It is imperative that students are prepared for all potential roles. Students may consult each other as the simulation exercise progresses. Accuracy needs to be ensured and students may choose to double-check the patient's vital signs and the medications being administered. The educator may reserve the right to grade students on an individual basis, especially if one member of the group is clearly unprepared for the exercise.

Simulation Grade

The educator will provide specific information related to the grading of the simulation exercise. The student's grade will be affected by the timely completion of skills with accuracy. The grading grid presented within this text recommends the following guidelines for grade construction.

1. Beginning Steps: (10%): This includes washing your hands, introducing yourself to the patient, explaining the plan of care, checking the proper patient identification (use two indicators), providing privacy, and donning gloves or applying the appropriate PPE as necessary. Students should understand the PPE requirements for a neutropenic patient.

2. Data Collection (30%): Prioritize data collection; recall the ABC's (airway, breathing, and circulation). Data collection should remain focused on key patient priorities. The first set of vital signs will be manual to ensure that students can accurately obtain an apical pulse, respirations, and blood pressure. Students should demonstrate the usage of all needed equipment. For example, to obtain the patients oxygen saturation correctly apply the device and wait for the educator to verbally provide the reading. The primary focus for this simulation exercise is end of life care. Be sure to review psychosocial aspects of patient care.

3. Implementation (30%): Performance of various nursing skills needs to be done in an accurate and timely manner. See the above information for content to review. Notification of the RN supervisor is required if the patient's status changes.

4. Evaluation (10%): Evaluate each intervention performed. After students perform an intervention they should question if the action resulted in the desired outcome; if not, formulation of other interventions may be required. Evaluate all medications administered. Re-check the patient's vital signs as this is required.

5. Postmortem Care (10%): Postmortem care discussion.

6. Student Professionalism (10%): Professional dress, proper communication, display of team work, preparedness for the scenario, and adaptation to stress will make up the final portion of the simulation grade.

Family Member Information

You came to the hospital with your mother and are upset with the rest of your family. They think that your mother should be moved to a hospice unit in town. You think she should die at home as she is requesting. You are the only sibling who feels this way. Your mother is a widow and has shared with you that she wants to die soon and be with your late father. She has a strong faith and feels it is time to go "home." There has been a great deal of arguing with your siblings about your mother and you are very tired of the drama. You have notified her priest to let him know how sick your mother is. You are tearful but remain close to your mom. The remainder of your family has been notified that she has been admitted to the hospital.

Case Study for Simulation 7
Cancer & End of Life (Adult)

1. Discuss neutropenic significance in this scenario.
2. Define symptoms of distress at the end of life.
3. Discuss goals for end of life care.
4. Describe postmortem care.
5. What are the signs and symptoms of the dying process?
6. The topic of death may be difficult. Discuss methods of coping used by the professional nurse in the event of a patient's death.
7. Chart on the end of life cares that you provided Jean Hafner per the educator's guidelines.

Data Collection & Medication Administration (Pediatric)

Goals/Outcomes of Simulation Exercise

- Students will demonstrate age-appropriate data collection and identify abnormal findings.
- Students will prioritize care and communicate abnormal findings to supervisor.
- Students will demonstrate age-appropriate medication administration.
- Students will verbalize age-appropriate communication techniques.

Acute Patient Information

It is the evening shift (1500) and students will provide care to Scotty Bauer, a 6-month-old male infant who was admitted to the pediatric unit 8 hours ago with a primary diagnosis of bacterial pneumonia and a secondary diagnosis of dehydration. Scotty's grandparent stated that he was diagnosed with pneumonia 3 days ago, was prescribed Zithromax, but was "getting worse rather than better." Upon admission the grandparent reported that Scotty had difficulty breathing, stating, "It was really fast." Scotty's liquid intake had decreased by 75% and he refused to eat any solid foods. The grandparent reported that Scotty had 2 wet diapers and several episodes of diarrhea in the 12 hours prior to admission. The grandparent observed that Scotty's buttocks region is very red and stated, "It looks like a yeast rash he had 2 months ago."

Scotty is now alert, makes eye contact, and reaches for objects. His admitting respiratory rate was 62 breaths per minute, and his admitting oxygen saturation was 88% on room air. The admitting nurse also reported these respiratory findings: a harsh productive cough, bilateral course crackles, intercostal retractions, use of accessory muscles, and nasal flaring. His clothing smelled of cigarette smoke. Upon admission Scotty's skin was pale, his capillary refill was 3 seconds, no tearing was observed with crying, and his mucous membranes were dry. The admitting nurse auscualted a heart murmur. An innocent heart murmur was previously noted within his clinic chart. An initial 140 mL intravenous (IV) bolus of sodium chloride (NaCl) was administered upon admission. Scotty's grandparent has been attentive and is encouraging oral fluid intake on a frequent basis. His mother could not be located for admission consent. Scotty has had two wet diapers in the past 7 hours. The admitting nurse agrees with the grandparent that Scotty potentially has a yeast rash on his buttocks and will notify the physician after report. He currently has a 22 gauge IV in his left saphenous vein with 0.9% NaCl infusing at a rate of 28 mL/hr.

At 1400 Scotty's vital signs were as follows: respirations 48 breaths per minute, apical pulse 146 beats per minute, tympanic temperature 101.6 °F, and oxygen saturation 96% on ½ liter of oxygen per nasal cannula. Scotty appears to be resting more comfortably now that his breathing has slowed. Admitting labs were as follows: white blood count (WBC) 22 μ/L, serum potassium (K+) 3.9 mmol/L, serum sodium (Na+) 141 mmol/L, blood cultures are pending. A chest x-ray showed consolidation in the bilateral lower lobes, greater on the right. Influenza and respiratory syncytial virus (RSV) tests were negative.

Other Relevant Patient Information

- Past medical diagnosis: otitis media, 2 months ago
- Prenatal history: five prenatal visits (all during the last trimester)
- Born at 38 weeks; weight 6 pounds 2 ounces
- Current weight 15.5 pounds
- Current length 25 inches
- Up to date on immunizations
- Current medications: Zithromax, third dose administered today at 0600 (prescription for five doses); the grandparent is unsure if the second dose was administered by the patient's mother
- Allergies: no known food or drug allergies

Guidelines for Student Preparation

Prior to the simulation exercise students should review the following medication list and prepare to perform the indicated skills. Be sure to read Chapter 1 of the student text for additional guidelines. As students review medications the following information should be noted: the trade and generic names, the indications of each medication, the safe dosage ranges, various routes of administration, primary nursing implications, and common side effects.

- Medications used within this simulation include: cefuroxime (IV), acetaminophen, ibuprofen, Xopenex nebulizer, and IV maintenance fluid of 0.9% sodium chloride (NaCl).
- Review dosage calculations prior to the simulation exercise as calculation will be required during medication administration. Understand how to calculate weight-based medication dosages for pediatrics.
- Students must be aware of IV considerations related to an infant (i.e. safe rates, monitoring of the IV site, and proper size of the IV bag).
- Students should be familiar with the procedure of administering a nebulizer treatment to a 6-month-old infant.
- Students should fully review the data collection process. Be aware that a patient chart will be available for review during the simulation exercise.
- Students should demonstrate how to manually obtain all patient vital signs including apical pulse, respirations, oxygen saturation, and temperature. Note that the simulated patient will be an infant. Know the normal range of infant vital signs.
- Students should understand how to assess an infant for signs and symptoms of respiratory distress. Human patient simulators may not be able to display signs such as nasal flaring and retractions. Students **MUST** be sure to verbalize when observing for signs of respiratory distress and be specific in order to gain patient data. For example, a student could

state, "I am observing for nasal flaring and use of accessory muscles." The educator will then provide information in regards to the assessed data. Points may be deducted if omission of respiratory data occurs.

- Application of oxygen to an infant patient should be reviewed.
- Students should review the process of giving a verbal report.
- Talk to the simulator as you would a "real" patient. Be sure to provide age appropriate care. Ask the grandparent questions as the educator will provide some of the verbal responses (some responses will be provided by the grandparent). Consider your approach to a 6-month-old and how you might alter care.
- Keep safety measures related to an infant in mind.
- Explain the plan of care to the grandparent. Provide education when administering medications or performing a procedure.
- Students must be able to understand the following lab values: serum potassium (K+), serum sodium (Na+), white blood cell count (WBC), and blood cultures.
- Students must demonstrate proper documentation of medications on the medication administration record (MAR). Students may be required to write a nurses note in relation to the simulation events. Information (i.e. vital signs) obtained during the simulation event should be recorded.

Student Simulation Roles

The student simulation roles are as follows: a team leader, medication nurse, data collection nurse, and family member (grandparent). The educator may choose to restructure roles as deemed necessary. For further review of the student roles refer to Chapter 1 of this text. Roles may be assigned just prior to the simulation exercise start. It is imperative that students are prepared for all potential roles. As this is a team effort students may consult each other as the simulation exercise progresses. Students may choose to double-check the patient's vital signs and the medications being administered. The educator may reserve the right to grade students on an individual basis, especially if one member of the team is clearly unprepared for the exercise.

Simulation Grade

The educator will provide specific information related to the grading of the simulation exercise. The student's grade will be affected by the timely completion of skills with accuracy. The grading grid presented within this text recommends the following guidelines for grade construction.

Case Study for Simulation 8 Data Collection & Medication Administration (Pediatric)

1. Scotty is diagnosed with bacterial pneumonia. Viral pneumonia is also common in infants. Discuss the differences between bacterial and viral pneumonia.
2. Discuss the signs and symptoms of respiratory decline in infants.
3. Discuss the safety precautions that the nurse must consider when caring for a pediatric patient receiving IV therapy.
4. What are the primary indications for cefuroxime? What is the dosage range of cefuroxime for infants (i.e. mg/kg)? What are common side effects that must be monitored for?
5. A red rash was observed by Scotty's grandparent and the admission nurse. A yeast rash is suspected. Discuss the risk factors for a yeast infection.
6. Several concerns relating to Scotty's social history arise during this simulation. What pieces of data are concerning? What is the PN's role in addressing these concerns?
7. Reflection is a vital part of the learning process. Discuss what went well during the simulation experience and what areas need improvement.
8. Chart on the care that you provided Scotty per the educator's guidelines.

Respiratory & Croup (Infant)

Goals/Outcomes of Simulation Exercise

- Students will demonstrate age appropriate data collection and report abnormal findings to the supervisor.
- Students will demonstrate age appropriate medication administration.
- Students will provide discharge teaching instructions related to croup.
- Students will verbalize age appropriate communication techniques.

Acute Patient Information

It is the day shift (0900) and students will provide care to Dylan Derheim, a 9-month-old male infant who presents to an urgent care clinic with his parent. Dylan's parent reports that he had a "barking cough" throughout the night. His parent states, "He still seems to be struggling to get air." No further data is provided because this patient is just arriving to the urgent care clinic. In this simulation scenario students will need to gather data directly from the patient and family member. The RN nursing supervisor (i.e., the educator) can be contacted as the need arises.

Other Relevant Patient Information

■ Past medical diagnosis: healthy; parent reports a "few colds"
■ Prenatal history: mother attended all recommended physician visits, uncomplicated pregnancy
■ Born at 39 weeks; weight 7 pounds 8 ounces
■ Parent unsure of current weight
■ Up to date on immunizations
■ Current medications: none
■ Breastfed; foods slowly being introduced
■ Allergies: no known food or drug allergies

Guidelines for Student Preparation

For student success, a review of the following medications and skills are required prior to the simulation exercise. Be sure to review Chapter 1 for further student guidelines. As students review medications the following information should be noted: the trade and generic name, the indications of the medications, the safe dosage ranges, primary nursing implications and the common side effects.

■ Medications used within this simulation include: oral acetaminophen, dexamethasone intramuscular (IM), and a cool mist nebulizer.
■ Students should review how to calculate medications based upon weight.
■ Students should fully review the data collection process. Understand what data might be normal or abnormal in an infant patient.
■ Students should review the process of giving a verbal report to the RN supervisor once data collection is complete.
■ Students should understand signs of infant respiratory distress. Human patient simulators may not be able to display signs such as nasal flaring and retractions. However, it is impetrative that the nurse monitors for such data. Students **MUST** be sure to state when observing for signs

of respiratory distress; be specific in order to gain patient data. For example, a student could state, "I am observing for nasal flaring and use of accessory muscles". The educator will then provide information in regards to the assessed data. Points may be deducted if omission of respiratory data occurs.

- Students should understand how to administer a cool mist nebulizer treatment to an infant.
- Student will be required to demonstrate how to obtain a full set of vital signs. Know normal vital sign parameters for a 9-month-old.
- Students will be required to verbally state how to obtain a weight on an infant patient.
- Students must understand the procedure of administering an intramuscular (IM) injection to an infant. Understand the proper landmarks and safety considerations. Team members should be sure to properly hold the HPS injection location to prevent the "infant" from "moving".
- Student will need to obtain sample swabs to test for respiratory syncytial virus (RSV) and influenza.
- Students must demonstrate therapeutic communication with the parent. Review the patient information above and pre-plan how you will comfort the parent in this situation. If a parent is very nervous this may increase the stress level of the infant.
- Educate the parent about the medical condition and interventions being performed.
- Students must demonstrate proper documentation of medications administered on the medication administration record (MAR). In addition, information during the simulation event such as vital signs should be recorded by students for later documentation.

Student Simulation Roles

The student simulation roles are as follows: team leader, medication nurse, data collection nurse, and family member. The educator may choose to restructure roles as deemed necessary. For further review of the student roles refer to Chapter 1 of the student text. Roles may be assigned just prior to the simulation exercise start. It is imperative that students are prepared for all potential roles. Students may consult each other as the simulation exercise progresses. Accuracy needs to be ensured and students may choose to double check the patients vital signs and the medications being administered. The educator may reserve the right to grade students on an individual basis especially if one member of the team is clearly unprepared for the exercise.

Simulation Grade

The educator will provide specific information related to the grading of the simulation exercise. The student's grade will be affected by the timely completion of skills with accuracy. The grading grid presented within this text recommends the following guidelines for grade construction.

1. Beginning Steps (5%): This includes handwashing, introducing one-self to the parent, and checking the patient identification band.

2. Data Collection (30%): Data collection should remain focused on key patient priorities. Vital signs will be manual to ensure that students can accurately obtain an apical pulse and respirations. Students should demonstrate the usage of all needed equipment. For example, to obtain the patients oxygen saturation, correctly apply the device and wait for the educator to verbally provide the reading. Respiratory status is the key focus of this simulation scenario and students should pre-plan how to focus data collection on the respiratory system. Hydration status of the infant is also a concern. Communication of any abnormal findings should occur in a timely fashion. Recall that a supervising RN will be available if needed.

3. Verbal Report (10%): Once the data collection is complete an update should be provided to the RN supervisor; this can be done by the team leader. Students should clearly communicate all data collection information. The certified nurse practitioner (CNP) will evaluate the patient and then provide written orders. *Students will not need to interact with the CNP; orders will "appear."*

4. Implementation (30%): Performance of nursing skills needs to be done in an accurate and timely manner. See the above information for content to review. Significant points may be deducted if a medication error is made. Students will need to administer a cool mist nebulizer, oral medications, and an IM medication. Students will need to obtain sample swabs as indicated above. Students should notify the lab and x-ray department of orders which need to be carried out. As you implement interventions provide age-appropriate care. Educate the parent on the plan of care.

5. Evaluation (10%): Evaluate each intervention performed. After students perform an intervention, question if the action resulted in the desired outcome. Evaluation for this simulation may include repeated vital signs, and re-evaluation of any abnormal findings.

6. Discharge (5%): Upon the conclusion of the simulation exercise students will be required to provide discharge instructions to the parent. The RN supervisor has written the discharge instructions and has delegated that students review the information with the

parent. The discharge should be clear, concise, and organized. Effective communication must be demonstrated.

7. Student Professionalism (10%): Professional dress, proper communication, display of teamwork, preparedness for the scenario, and adaptation to stress will make up the final portion of the simulation grade.

Family Member Information

> **Note to student assigned the family role:** This is an anxious time for you. Insist on touching, kissing, and providing comfort to your child.

You arrive at the urgent care clinic with your son Dylan. He had a harsh barking cough and all night and couldn't breathe normally. Dylan did seem to get slightly better in the car (as he was exposed to the cool air outside), but this was only temporary. Dylan is typically healthy and is cared for at home. Dylan has been fussy and has not been nursing well for the past two days. He refused to nurse at bedtime last night. He has had a runny nose and has not been able to sleep well for two days. You have a 4-year-old son at home named Tyler and wonder if he will get sick too.

The student playing the role of the family member should be sure to ask the nurses many questions.

Case Study for Simulation 9
Respiratory & Croup (Infant)

1. Dylan is diagnosed by the nurse practitioner with croup. Dylan's parent does not know what croup is. How would you describe this condition?

2. How should the nurse tailor data collection in regards to the diagnosis of croup? What are the key points of information to observe?

3. When reviewing the lab results presented earlier in this chapter, a high lymphocyte and low neutrophil count are observed. What might this indicate? Why might this be important information in the treatment?

4. Dexamethasone was ordered for this patient. Why might it be indicated?

5. Are patients diagnosed with croup able to go home? What might the criteria be for hospital admission?

6. When providing the parent education in regards to acetaminophen administration, what key points should the nurse stress?

7. The parent questioned if this condition will affect Dylan's 4-year-old sibling Tyler. How might the nurses respond to this question?

8. Reflection is a vital part of the learning process. Discuss what went well during the simulation experience and what areas need improvement.

9. Chart on the care you provided Dylan Derheim per the educator's guidelines.

Endocrine & Diabetes (Pediatric)

Goals/Outcomes of Simulation Exercise

- Students will demonstrate age-appropriate data collection and report abnormal findings.
- Students will calculate an insulin dose based on carbohydrate consumption.
- Students will allow the patient to express concerns and fear in regard to diabetic diagnosis.

Acute Patient Information

It is the day shift (0700) and students will provide care to Sarah Holt, a 12-year-old female patient who was transferred to the medical unit two days ago from the intensive care unit with a primary diagnosis of diabetic ketoacidosis. Sarah presented to the emergency department (ED) three days ago after her family found her unresponsive. History per the ED note includes polydipsia and polyuria. Lab urinalysis revealed a urinary tract infection (UTI). Her last dose of antibiotic was given yesterday. The family reports that Sarah had flu-like symptoms including nausea, vomiting, and abdominal pain two days prior to admission.

Sarah is quiet and orientated to person, place, and time. The night nurse reports that she has not been talking much and does not make eye contact with the nursing staff. Sarah has been arguing with her parent and is uncooperative. Her last set of vital signs at 0600 was 22 respirations per minute, apical pulse regular at 72 beats per minute, blood pressure 98/64, tympanic temperature 98.9 °F, and oxygen saturation 99% on room air.

Her initial admission labs were blood glucose 650 mg/dL, serum potassium (K+) 4.8 mEq/L, white blood cell count (WBC) 12.2 μ/L, serum pH 7.20, serum HCO_3 12 mEq/L, BUN 22 mEq/L, urine ketones were positive, and urine tested positive for white and red cells. Lab results at 0600 were blood glucose 84 mg/dL, K+ 3.4 mEq/L, serum pH 7.39, serum HCO_3 15.2 mEq/L, BUN 18, and urine ketones were negative.

Sarah's skin is warm, dry, and pale. Weight is 170 this morning. Lungs are clear and heart tones are normal. Capillary refill time is 3 seconds. She has a 20 gauge saline lock (SL) in her left forearm.

Sarah lives with her parent and two younger brothers. She has been involved in music at school but has avoided any sport activities. Her parent says she spends "too much time" in front of the computer and TV and does not spend much time with friends. She is withdrawn from family activities. Her father and mother divorced three years ago, and she does not see her other parent more than once or twice a year.

Other Relevant Patient Information

- Admission diagnosis: diabetic ketoacidosis with new diagnosis of type 1 diabetes, UTI, and depression
- Past history of polydipsia, polyuria
- Height 4'8"
- Admission weight 174 lbs
- Current home medications: none
- Allergies: none

Guidelines for Student Preparation

Prior to the simulation exercise students should review the following medication list and prepare to perform the indicated skills. Be sure to read Chapter 1 of the student text for additional guidelines. As students review medications the following information should be noted: the trade and generic names, the indications of each medication, safe dosage ranges, various routes of administration, primary nursing implications, and common side effects.

- Medications used within this simulation include: Lantus and Humalog insulin, Zoloft, and a saline lock flush.
- Students will need to understand carbohydrate calculation and corresponding insulin dosage. The breakfast tray will consist of: two pieces of wheat toast, 1/2 banana, one carton of skim milk, and sugar-free jam.
- Students should fully review the data collection process. Be aware that a patient chart will be available for review during the simulation exercise.
- Students should be able to demonstrate how to manually obtain all patient vital signs including blood pressure, apical pulse, respirations, oxygen saturation, and temperature.
- Students must verbalize therapeutic communication.
- Students should educate the patient on the medications administered during the simulation exercise.
- Students should be familiar with the procedure of flushing a saline lock (SL).
- Students must demonstrate obtaining a capillary blood glucose reading.
- Students must be able to understand the following lab values: blood glucose, electrolyte panel, CBC, arterial blood gases, and urine ketones.
- Students must demonstrate proper documentation of medications on the medication administration record (MAR). Students may be required to document simulation events at the discretion of the educator. Information during the simulation event should be recorded.
- Students should be prepared to notify the RN supervisor in regard to patient condition changes.

Student Simulation Roles

The student simulation roles are as follows: team leader, medication nurse, data collection nurse, and family member. The educator may choose to restructure roles as deemed necessary. For further review of the student roles refer to chapter one of the student text. Roles may be assigned prior to the simulation exercise start. It is imperative that students are prepared for all potential roles. Students may consult each other as the simulation exercise progresses. Accuracy needs to be ensured and students may choose to double-check the patient's vital signs and the medications being administered.

Student must recall pediatric guidelines for medication administration. The educator may reserve the right to grade students on an individual basis, especially if one member of the team is clearly unprepared for the exercise.

Simulation Grade

The educator will provide specific information related to the grading of the simulation exercise. The student's grade will be affected by the timely completion of skills with accuracy. The grading grid presented within this text recommends the following guidelines for grade construction.

1. Beginning Steps (10%): This includes washing your hands, introducing yourself to the patient, explaining the plan of care, checking the proper patient identification (use two indicators), providing privacy, and donning gloves or applying the appropriate PPE as necessary (i.e. when checking capillary blood glucose).

2. Data Collection (30%): Prioritize data collection; recall the ABC's (airway, breathing, and circulation). Data collection should remain focused on key priorities in regard to the diabetic patient. The first set of vital signs will be taken manually to ensure that students can accurately obtain an apical pulse, respirations, and blood pressure. Students should demonstrate the usage of all needed equipment. Calculation of carbohydrate intake is necessary for insulin dosage. Students should be sure to assess the patient's psychosocial status.

3. Implementation (30%): Performance of various nursing skills needs to be done in an accurate and timely manner. See the above information for content to review. Within this section, students will be required to administer some of the medications listed above. Significant points may be deducted for medication errors. Students must demonstrate the administration of short and long acting insulin. Students must perform a saline lock flush.

4. Evaluation (10%): Evaluate each intervention performed. After students perform an intervention, question if the action resulted in the desired outcome. Evaluate the medications administered to determine if the desired effect of the medication occurred. This may include rechecking the patient's capillary blood glucose.

5. Verbal Report (10%): During the simulation exercise students will be required to provide a verbal report to the RN supervisor and address all of the concerns that arise during the simulation exercise. The verbal report should be clear, concise, and organized. Effective communication must be demonstrated.

6. Student Professionalism (10%): Professional dress, proper communication, display of teamwork, preparedness for the scenario, and adaptation to stress will make up the final portion of the simulation grade.

Family Member Information

Sarah has been more withdrawn at home and is spending additional time in her room. Her parent states she does not find pleasure in activities that she normally enjoys. Her behavior has changed drastically in the past two months. Fighting between Sarah and her brothers has escalated in the past two weeks. Her change in behavior has been difficult for the family. Her parent describes her as depressed and tearful. Sarah's parent further states concern that her school grades have dropped during the past month.

Case Study for Simulation 10
Endocrine & Diabetes (Pediatric)

1. In a table format, describe the differences between hypoglycemia and hyperglycemia.

2. Sarah presents with the initial diagnosis of diabetic ketoacidosis. Which findings in her history, lab report, and exam support this diagnosis?

3. What is the expected action the student will take to prevent a hypoglycemic reaction?

4. With the noted psychosocial history for Sarah, what types of psychosocial interventions would the student use in conversation with Sarah?

5. The RN has outlined a teaching plan for Sarah in regard to her diabetes. One of the topics of teaching is diet therapy. Discuss the goals of diet therapy for Sarah.

6. Reflection is a vital part of the learning process. Discuss what went well during the simulation experience, and what areas need improvement.

7. Chart on the care that you provided Sarah per the educator's guidelines.

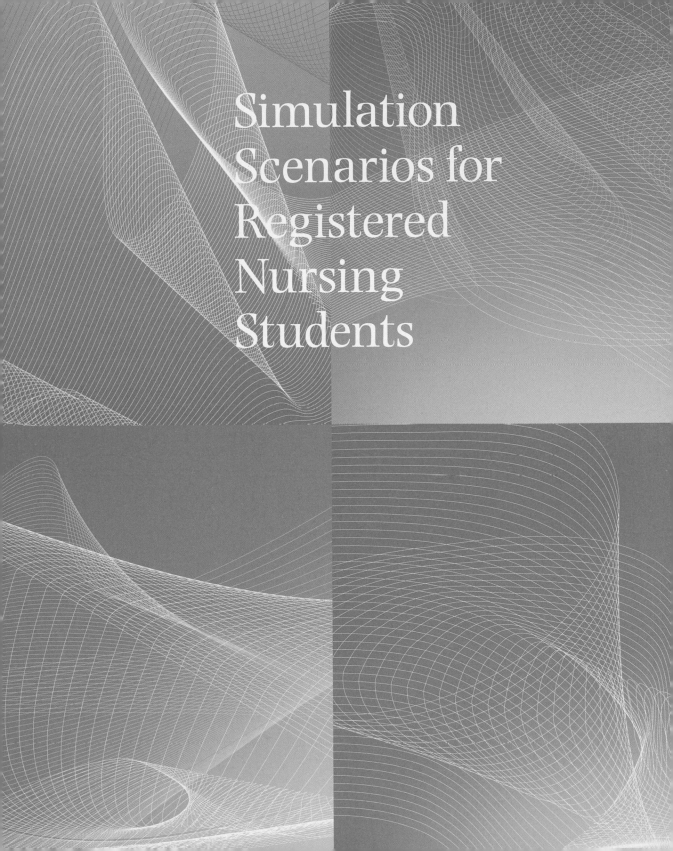

Simulation Scenarios for Registered Nursing Students

Assessment & Medication Administration (Adult)

Goals/Outcomes of Simulation Exercise

- Students will demonstrate a comprehensive assessment and identify abnormal findings.
- Students will demonstrate safe oral and intravenous (IV) medication administration.
- Students will demonstrate the skill component of inserting an indwelling urinary catheter.
- Students will verbalize pertinent patient information to a primary health care provider.

Acute Patient Information

It is the day shift (0700) and students will provide care to William Hampton, a 78-year-old male patient admitted to the medical unit two days ago with a primary diagnosis of congestive heart failure (CHF). William presented to his primary physician's clinic with a two day history of weakness, shortness of breath, and difficulty ambulating more than 10 feet. He reports that he has been unable to get out of bed for the past two days. A comparison of William's weight from a previous visit two weeks ago indicated an 11 pound weight increase. William reports that he rarely needs his PRN oxygen but has used it continuously for the past two days.

William is alert and orientated to person, place, and time. The night nurse reports that his respirations were 38 breaths per minute with ambulation to the bathroom. The nurse counseled him to use a urinal for energy conservation but recommends that an indwelling urinary catheter may be needed. William rested off and on throughout the night, voiding a total of 400 mL. His last set of vital signs at 0530 was: 26 respirations/minute at rest; apical pulse irregular 92 beats/minute; blood pressure 118/70; tympanic temperature 99.5 °F and oxygen saturation 91% on 2 liters of oxygen per nasal cannula. William denies any pain or discomfort. The 0630 lab results are as follows: B-type natriuretic peptide (BNP) 2300 pg/mL; serum potassium (K+) 4.2 mEq/L; and white blood cell count (WBC) 16.2 μ/L. The night nurse states that she has not had time to call the physician and inform him of the lab values because the results posted 10 minutes ago. She requested that the day shift notify Dr. Uselman after report in regard to the lab values and request for a urinary catheter. William has a 20 gauge saline lock (SL) in his left forearm; no intravenous (IV) fluids are infusing at this time.

Bilateral course crackles were auscultated by the night nurse. William has a frequent productive cough of clear sputum. His bowel sounds are active and he reports feeling hungry for breakfast. The night nurse reported 3+ pitting edema bilaterally in William's ankles and feet. Pedal pulses were difficult to palpate. The night nurse stated that "the ordered TED hose (anti-embolism stockings) will be next to impossible to put on; an order other than TED hose should be obtained when the physician is notified." As of this morning William's weight is down six pounds since his admission two days ago. William slept with the head of the bed elevated 45 degrees.

William lives alone. He speaks frequently of his late wife who died two years ago; they had been married for 55 years. Many grandchildren take turns visiting him daily. He is now considering getting a pet to help decrease the feeling of being alone in an empty house. William enjoys talking about current events and frequently watches various news channels on TV. The night nurse jokes, "I hope you are up to date on current events" as she leaves for the day. Students will begin care of William at 0730.

Other Relevant Patient Information

- Medical diagnoses: CHF, atrial fibrillation, chronic obstructive pulmonary disease (COPD), hypertension (HTN), and hypothyroidism
- Past history of smoking: began smoking at the age of 14, quit 10 years ago
- Height 6'0"
- Morning weight today 235 pounds
- Current medications—all medications are via the oral route unless indicated otherwise: multivitamin one daily, Colace 100 mg daily, Synthroid 75 mcg daily, Coreg 25 mg twice a day, Lasix 40 mg IV push twice a day, K-Dur 20 mEq twice a day, digoxin 0.25 mg daily, Zestril 10 mg daily, ASA EC 81 mg daily, Zithromax 250 mg daily, Advair 250/50 one puff twice a day, and albuterol nebulizer 1 unit dose every 4–6 hours as needed.
- Allergies: sulfa

Guidelines for Student Preparation

For student success, a review of the following medications and skills are required prior to the simulation exercise. Be sure to read Chapter 1 of the student text for additional guidelines. As students review medications the following information should be noted: the trade and generic names, the indications of each medication, safe dosage ranges, primary nursing implications, and common side effects. Students should review the rate at which to administer the ordered IV push medication.

- Review pre-steps to patient care: handwashing, introduction of self to the patient, verifying patient identification via two identifiers (name & date of birth), ensuring privacy, and utilization of gloves and personal protective equipment (PPE) when necessary.
- Students should fully review the assessment process. The ability to conduct a comprehensive assessment will be required. The assessment nurse should share any abnormal assessment findings with the supervisor.
- Students should be able to demonstrate how to manually obtain all patient vital signs including blood pressure, apical pulse, respirations, oxygen saturation, and temperature. Understand the HPS functions to increase competency of these skills.
- Students must demonstrate therapeutic communication with the patient and family member. Speak to the HPS and ask questions. The educator will provide patient responses.
- Medications used within this simulation include: multivitamin, Colace, Synthroid, Coreg, Lasix (IV push), K-Dur, digoxin, Zestril, ASA, Zithromax, Advair, albuterol nebulizer, and a saline lock flush.

- Students should educate the patient in regard to the medications being administered and procedures being performed during the simulation exercise. Students should also educate the patient in regard to his medical condition.
- Students should review dosage calculations prior to the simulation exercise, as they will be required during medication administration.
- Students should be familiar with the procedure of flushing a saline lock (SL).
- Students should be prepared to administer an albuterol nebulizer as it is a PRN medication. Students should also understand when this medication would be indicated.
- Students should review the application of oxygen via various methods.
- Students must be able to understand the following lab values: B-type natriuretic peptide (BNP), serum potassium, and white blood cell count (WBC). Students will need to call the health care provider and report these results.
- Students must demonstrate proper documentation of medications on the medication administration record (MAR). Information during the simulation event (i.e. vital signs) should be recorded as the educator may later require documentation of the simulation exercise.
- Students should be prepared to notify the health care provider in regard to the patient condition and understand the process for receiving verbal orders via phone. A phone will be provided in the simulation environment.
- Students should be familiar with the application of ACE wraps (elastic bandages) to reduce swelling to the lower extremities.
- Students should be familiar with the insertion of an indwelling urinary catheter.

Hint:
Consider what assessment information the health care provider may want to know in addition to the lab values.

Student Simulation Roles

The student simulation roles are as follows: supervisor, medication nurse, assessment nurse, and family member. The educator may choose to restructure roles as deemed necessary. For further review of the student roles refer to Chapter 1 of the student text. Roles may be assigned prior to the simulation exercise start. It is imperative that students are prepared for all potential roles. As this is a team effort, students may consult each other as the simulation exercise progresses. Accuracy needs to be ensured and students may choose to double-check the patient's vital signs and the medications being administered. Please note that the educator may reserve the right to grade students on an individual basis, especially if one member of the team is clearly unprepared for the exercise.

Simulation Grade

The educator will provide specific information related to the grading of the simulation exercise. The student's grade will be affected by the timely completion of skills with accuracy. If this is the first simulation exercise students have participated in, the grading grid may be followed with the final evaluation resulting in a pass or fail. The grading grid presented within this text recommends the following guidelines for grade construction.

1. Beginning Steps (10%): This includes washing your hands, introducing yourself to the patient, explaining the plan of care, checking the proper patient identification (use two indicators), providing privacy, and donning gloves or applying the appropriate PPE as necessary.

2. Assessment (30%): Prioritize the assessment; recall the ABC's (airway, breathing, and circulation). The assessment should remain focused on key patient priorities. The vital signs will be manual to ensure that students can accurately obtain an apical pulse, respirations, and blood pressure. Students should demonstrate the usage of all needed equipment. For example, to obtain the patient's oxygen saturation, correctly apply the device and wait for the educator to verbally provide the reading. Students should further expand upon the patient information learned in report. Subjective and objective data should be assessed. The assessment should include inspection of the anterior and posterior HPS surfaces. Take care not to damage the HPS while turning it.

3. Verbal Report (10%): During the simulation exercise students will be required to provide an update of the patient's condition to the primary physician. Students should report pertinent patient information relayed from the previous shift and any concerning assessment findings. The verbal report should be clear, concise, and organized. Effective communication must be demonstrated. Students should understand the process for receiving verbal physician orders.

4. Implementation (30%): Performance of various nursing skills needs to be done in an accurate and timely manner. See the above information indicating skills to review. Students will be required to administer some of the medications listed above. Be sure to review all guidelines of medication administration listed in Chapter 1. Dosage calculation must be performed within this simulation. If a question arises during medication administration, inform the supervisor, who will address the issue. Significant points may be deducted for medication errors. Students should implement verbal orders received from the physician.

5. Evaluation (10%): Students should evaluate each nursing intervention. The patient's response to each performed action should be analyzed. If the desired outcome was not achieved, formulation of other interventions may be required. Evaluate medications administered to determine if the desired effect of the medication occurred. Reassessment of vital signs is required.

6. Student Professionalism (10%): Professional dress, proper communication, display of teamwork, preparedness for the scenario, and adaptation to stress will make up the final portion of the simulation grade.

Family Member Information

Your grandfather is a very kind man. He lives alone. You are from a large family and he does receive daily visits from family members. The family has discussed aiding him in obtaining a pet as suggested by his family physician. He complained about an increase in weakness and difficulty ambulating a few days ago, so another relative brought him in for an evaluation, after which point he was admitted to the hospital. He does try to follow most of his doctor's recommendations. However, he eats a lot of canned soup and processed foods high in salt. You feel that he does this for ease of meal preparation. Your grandfather is mentally sharp because he "always keeps his mind going with current events." In fact, you would say that you get a great deal of information regarding current events from him.

Case Study for Simulation 1
Assessment & Medication Administration (Adult)

1. Heart failure is described in literature as either right- or left-sided. Make a comparison table comparing the signs and symptoms of right- and left-sided heart failure.

2. Crackles were noted bilaterally in Mr. Hampton's lungs. Describe what crackles indicate and what further assessment criteria should be evaluated.

3. During the simulation exercise, it was discovered that the certified nursing assistant removed Mr. Hampton's oxygen and forgot to reapply it. What points of information will you include to provide further education to the CNA?

4. This simulation exercise had multiple medications ordered to lower Mr. Hampton's blood pressure. Which medications were administered for this purpose, and why are several medications ordered?

5. In report you learned that Mr. Hampton's BNP was 2300. Why was this information important for the night nurse to note?

6. Reflection is a vital part of the learning process. Discuss what went well during the simulation experience, and what areas need improvement.

7. Chart on the care that you provided Mr. Hampton per the educator's guidelines.

Urinary & Pyelonephritis (Adult)

Goals/Outcomes of Simulation Exercise

- Students will identify pertinent assessment findings and prioritize plan of care.
- Students will demonstrate skill components of intravenous (IV) medication administration and urine specimen collection.
- Students will provide a teaching plan on urinary tract infection prevention and safe sexual practices.
- Students will validate guidelines related to narcotic administration.

Acute Patient Information

It is the evening shift (1500) and students will provide care to Nanna Krause, a 21-year-old female patient who was just admitted with a primary diagnosis of pyelonephritis. Nanna reports that she began having signs and symptoms of a urinary tract infection five days ago. Nanna states she experienced a burning sensation with urination, had mild abdominal pain, and frequent urgent urination. She states, "I seriously had to go every 10 minutes." Nanna was advised by her good friend to take cranberry capsules, vitamin C tablets, and phenazopyridine. She began taking the medications after she researched them on the Internet because "they seemed to be what I needed." Nanna awoke this morning with a high fever, vomiting, and severe abdominal pain. Nanna further adds that she has moderate bilateral flank pain.

Nanna reports that she started having frequent urinary tract infections about the time she began college. She stated, "I know what they feel like." She vomited in the emergency department two hours ago. Nanna has a 20 gauge IV in her left hand with 0.9% sodium chloride (NaCl) infusing at 250 mL/hr. She has refused any oral intake. She voided 50 mL of cloudy, foul smelling, dark amber urine in the emergency department. Her last set of vital signs at 1400 were: respirations 14 per minute at rest; regular apical pulse 90 per minute; blood pressure 124/70; tympanic temperature 104.3 °F and oxygen saturation 98% on room air. She was given 1,000 mg of Tylenol in the emergency room for fever an hour ago.

The admitting lab results were as follows: pregnancy text negative, white blood cell count (WBC) 22.0 μL, blood urea nitrogen (BUN) 24 mg/dL, and gonorrhea and chlamydia cultures are pending. Nanna's urinalysis results were as follows: + red blood cells, + white blood cells, and + nitrites. The physician has ordered a mini catheterization to be done to obtain a sample for a urine culture. Medication orders have been sent to the pharmacy, and the IV antibiotics should be started after the mini catheterization.

Nanna's lung sounds are clear and her heart tones are regular. Bowel sounds are present. Her last bowel movement was yesterday and was reported to be "normal." Her abdomen is soft and tender to palpation. Pedal pulses are present and strong. Morphine 4 mg IV was administered in the emergency department (ED) one hour ago. She last rated her pain at 2 of 5 and stated, "The morphine really helped."

Other Relevant Patient Information

■ Past medical diagnosis: three urinary tract infections in the past year
■ Past history of smoking: began two years ago, smokes a few cigarettes on the weekends "when she goes out"
■ Alcohol intake: five to six beers on Friday and Saturday nights

- Frequent sexual activity with no use of birth control
- Height 5'5"
- Weight 125 pounds
- Current medications: cranberry capsules two twice a day, vitamin C tablets one tablet twice a day, and phenazopyridine. She states, "I can't remember if that one was once or twice a day" in reference to the phenazopyridine. The patient is uncertain of any of the medication dosages; no routine medications
- Allergies: none

Guidelines for Student Preparation

For student success, a review of the following medications and skills are required prior to the simulation exercise. Be sure to review Chapter 1 for further student guidelines. As students review medications the following information should be noted: the trade and generic names, the indications of each medication, safe dosage ranges, primary nursing implications, and common side effects.

- Medications used within this simulation include: morphine (IV), Vicodin (oral), ciprofloxacin (IV), Zofran (IV), and 0.9% sodium chloride (NaCl).
- Students should be sure to review the specific considerations of each IV push medication above. Students will also be required to administer a secondary IV medication (ciprofloxacin).
- Students should be familiar with specific considerations of narcotic administration.
- Students should fully review the assessment process. Review the provided patient chart during the simulation exercise.
- Student will be required to demonstrate how to obtain a full set of vital signs.
- Students will be required to demonstrate a mini catheterization.
- Students must verbalize therapeutic communication with the HPS. Review the patient information above. Pre-plan how you provide education on the topics identified in the patient history and the friend.
- Students should review the process of giving a verbal report upon the conclusion of the simulation exercise.
- Students must demonstrate proper documentation of medications on the medication administration record (MAR). Information during the simulation event, such as vital signs, should be recorded by students for later documentation.

Student Simulation Roles

The student simulation roles are as follows: supervisor, medication nurse, assessment nurse, and family member. The educator may choose to restructure roles as deemed necessary. For further review of the student roles refer to Chapter 1 of the student text. Roles may be assigned prior to the simulation exercise start. It is imperative that students are prepared for all potential roles. Students may consult each other as the simulation exercise progresses. Accuracy needs to be ensured and students may choose to double-check the patient's vital signs and the medications being administered. The educator may reserve the right to grade students on an individual basis, especially if one member of the team is clearly unprepared for the exercise.

Simulation Grade

The educator will provide specific information related to the grading of the simulation exercise. The student's grade will be affected by the timely completion of skills with accuracy. The grading grid presented within this text recommends the following guidelines for grade construction.

1. Beginning Steps (10%): This includes washing hands, introducing yourself to the patient, explaining the plan of care, checking the proper patient identification (use two indicators), providing privacy, and donning gloves or applying the appropriate personal protective equipment (PPE) as necessary.
2. Assessment (30%): Prioritize the patient assessment. The assessment should remain focused on key patient priorities. Vital signs will be taken manually to ensure that students can accurately obtain an apical pulse and respirations. Students should demonstrate the usage of all needed equipment. For example, to obtain the patient's oxygen saturation, correctly apply the device and wait for the educator to verbally provide the reading. Subjective and objective data should be gathered. Be sure to assess the patient's psychosocial history.
3. Implementation (30%): Performance of various nursing skills needs to be done in an accurate and timely manner. See the above information for content to review. Significant points may be deducted if a medication error is made. Students will be required to administer IV push medications, perform a mini catheterization, and begin an IV antibiotic. It is expected that students provide the HPS education related to: (a) urinary tract infection prevention, and (b) safe

sexual practices. Students should pre-plan information for patient education.

4. Evaluation (10%): Evaluate each intervention performed. After students perform an intervention they should question if the action resulted in the desired outcome. Evaluation for this simulation may include repeated vital signs, pain status, and assessment of patient education.

5. Verbal Report (10%): Upon the conclusion of the simulation exercise students will be required to provide a verbal report to the nurse who will continue patient care. The verbal report should be clear, concise, and organized. Effective communication must be demonstrated.

6. Student Professionalism (10%): Professional dress, proper communication, display of teamwork, preparedness for the scenario, and adaptation to stress will make up the final portion of the simulation grade.

Family Member Information (Friend)

You brought Nanna to the emergency room. The two of you have been friends since high school. Though you consider Nanna a great friend you are really worried about the choices she has begun to make now that she is away from home. She parties all night Friday and Saturday. She typically drinks heavy amounts of alcohol on the weekends. She used to be a star athlete in high school, especially in track and field. She has begun to smoke, which is something that she was opposed to in high school. Nanna has begun to have "adult relationships" with multiple men, of which you do not approve. You pull a nurse aside and ask her to speak to Nanna about the risk of pregnancy and sexually transmitted diseases. Nanna might listen to a professional about this topic. You have tried to discuss this topic with her in the past but are "just too embarrassed."

Case Study for Simulation 2
Urinary & Pyelonephritis (Adult)

1. Nanna reports taking cranberry capsules, vitamin C tablets, and phenazopyridine. Why might these medications be helpful to patients who have a urinary tract infection (UTI)?

2. What are the risk factors for urinary tract infections?

3. List three priority nursing diagnoses for Nanna.

4. Nanna's increased sexual activity correlates with frequent UTIs. Why might sexual activity increase Nanna's risk of a UTI? How can this risk be reduced?

5. Narcotics are administered within this simulation exercise. What actions should the nurse take if the narcotic count is incorrect?

6. Reflection is a vital part of the learning process. Discuss what went well during the simulation experience, and what areas need improvement.

7. Chart on the care that you provided Nanna per the educator's guidelines.

Orthopedic Surgery & Pulmonary Embolism (Adult)

Goals/Outcomes of Simulation Exercise

- Students will identify abnormal assessment findings related to the respiratory system.
- Students will initiate and prioritize nursing interventions in response to assessment findings.
- Students will calculate and initiate an intravenous (IV) heparin drip.
- Students will verbalize the plan of care with the patient and family.

Acute Patient Information

It is the day shift (0700) and students will provide care to Patrick Hand-lon, a 53-year-old male who had a left total knee replacement three days ago. Today he will be discharged home. He has a history of osteoarthritis in both knees. Postoperative progress has been considered normal up to this point. Physical and occupational therapy have conducted a discharge evaluation, and he is ready to be discharged home. Patrick uses a continuous passive motion (CPM) machine three to four times a day. His pain is controlled with two hydrocodone/acetaminophen tablets every four to six hours. Estimated blood loss during surgery was 400 mL. Patrick's hemoglobin today was 9.2 g/dL (stated in labs information later in this scenario). Significant ecchymosis is reported in the entire left leg from the thigh to ankle. He has an anti-embolism stocking on the right leg. A dressing has been applied over the left knee incision and an ACE (elastic) wrap covers the dressing down to his mind calf region.

Patrick is irritable and anxious to go home. He was restless throughout the night shift. Hydroxyzine was administered in addition to the hydrocodone/acetaminophen to keep pain at a "1–2" on a scale of 0–5 for the night nurse. At 0600 vital signs were as follows: blood pressure 172/98; apical pulse 72 per minute; respirations 22 per minute; tympanic temperature of 99.8 °F and oxygen saturation 94% on room air. The 0600 lab results were as follows: white blood cell count (WBC) 11 μL, hemoglobin (Hgb) 9.2 g/dL, and hematocrit (Hct) 25%. He has an 18 gauge saline lock in the right hand.

Patrick's lung sounds are diminished but clear. He had a large bowel movement early this morning. He complains of a poor appetite. He needs to be reminded to use his incentive spirometer, tells the nurses he is not interested in it, and states, "Quit bothering me about it." He refused to ambulate to the bathroom during the night and used a urinal. Equal bilateral pedal pulses are palpated. Edema is observed in the left lower leg and is rated at a 3+.

Patrick has been awake on and off all night and became more restless toward morning. He states that he is "a little short on air." The night nurse reports he was last medicated for pain at 0300. Students will begin care of Patrick at 0730.

Other Relevant Patient Information

- Height 5'11"
- Weight 210 pounds
- Previous medical diagnoses include: hypertension, gastric reflux

- Current medications: hydrochlorothiazide (HCTZ) 25 mg daily, Protonix 40 mg daily, hydrocodone/acetaminophen 7.5/500 mg 1–2 tablets every 4 hours PRN knee pain, hydroxyzine 25 mg every 4 hours PRN nausea, Colace 100 mg twice daily, multivitamin daily, and Coumadin 5 mg daily
- Allergies: penicillin (PCN)

Guidelines for Student Preparation

For student success, a review of the following medications and skills are required prior to the simulation exercise. Be sure to review Chapter 1 for further student guidelines. As students review medications the following information should be noted: the trade and generic names, the indications of each medication, the safe dosage ranges, primary nursing implications, and common side effects.

- Medications used within this simulation include: hydrochlorothiazide (HCTZ), Protonix, multivitamin, hydrocodone/acetaminophen, hydroxyzine, Coumadin, heparin (IV push), and heparin (IV drip).
- Intravenous (IV) push medications such as saline and heparin are required for this simulation exercise. Calculation of the heparin IV drip will be necessary. A saline lock flush will be required.
- Students should fully review the assessment process. Be aware that a patient chart will be available for review during the simulation exercise.
- Students should be able to demonstrate how to manually obtain all patient vital signs including blood pressure, apical pulse, respirations, oxygen saturation, and temperature.
- Students should review the application of oxygen via various methods.
- Students must demonstrate proper assessment technique related to the patient pain and respiratory status.
- Students should be able to evaluate changes in the patient's condition during the scenario.
- Students should review the process associated with providing a comprehensive verbal report to a healthcare provider.
- Students must verbalize therapeutic communication.
- Students must be able to understand the following lab values: white blood cell count (WBC), hemoglobin (Hgb), hematocrit (Hct), partial thromboplastin time (PTT), and pro-time (PT).
- Students should understand the process involved in obtaining verbal physician's orders via telephone. A blank physician's order sheet will be present in the patient chart.
- Students must demonstrate proper documentation of medications on the medication administration record (MAR). Students may be required to write a nursing note in relation to the simulation events.

Student Simulation Roles

The student simulation roles are as follows: a supervisor, medication nurse, assessment nurse, and family member. The educator may choose to restructure roles as deemed necessary. For further review of the student roles refer to Chapter 1 of this text. Roles may be assigned prior to the simulation exercise start. It is imperative that students are prepared for all potential roles. Students may consult each other as the simulation exercise progresses. Accuracy needs to be ensured and students may choose to double-check the patient's vital signs and the medications being administered. The educator may reserve the right to grade students on an individual basis, especially if one member of the group is clearly unprepared for the exercise.

Simulation Grade

The educator will provide specific information related to the grading of the simulation exercise. The student's grade will be affected by the timely completion of skills with accuracy. The grading grid presented within this text recommends the following guidelines for grade construction.

1. Beginning Steps: (10%): This includes washing your hands, introducing yourself to the patient, explaining the plan of care, checking the proper patient identification (use two indicators), providing privacy, and donning gloves or applying the appropriate PPE as necessary.

2. Assessment (30%): Prioritize the patient assessment; recall the ABC's (airway, breathing, and circulation). The assessment should remain focused on key patient priorities. The first set of vital signs will be taken manually to ensure that students can accurately obtain an apical pulse, respirations, and blood pressure. Students should demonstrate the usage of all needed equipment. For example, to obtain the patient's oxygen saturation correctly, apply the device and wait for the educator to verbally provide the reading. As students assess the patient, formulate nursing diagnoses and plan interventions to implement. The primary focus for this simulation exercise is pain evaluation and respiratory status. Students will need to perform a focused assessment and react accordingly to changes in condition.

3. Report (10%): Students will need to call the primary care provider and report changes in patient status. Verbal orders will be given and students should be prepared to take verbal orders over the phone. Prior to calling the health care provider, make sure

all pertinent patient information is assessed. It is the role of the supervisor to call the health care provider.

4. Implementation (30%): Performance of various nursing skills needs to be done in an accurate and timely manner. See the above information of content to review. Be sure to implement the physician orders in a timely fashion. Students should communicate with other departments (i.e. lab, EKG, and x-ray) any physician's orders which need to be carried out.

5. Evaluation (10%): Evaluate each intervention performed. After students perform an action they should question if the action resulted in the desired outcome; if not, formulation of other interventions may be required. Evaluate all medications administered. Re-check the patient's vital signs as this is required.

6. Student Professionalism (10%): Professional dress, proper communication, display of teamwork, preparedness for the scenario, and adaptation to stress will make up the final portion of the simulation grade.

Family Member Information

Patrick is used to being very active but has had increased knee pain over the last six months. He is a teacher at an elementary school and hopes that this surgery will help with his activity level. He is married and has three grown children and three grandchildren. As the family member, you are concerned that he will do more than he is supposed to do at home. He is very stubborn and at times non-compliant when it comes to his heath care. When you came today to take him home he seemed to be much more agitated. You wonder what may have occurred. You are worried about his pain level and concerned how you will help care for him at home.

Case Study for Simulation 3 Orthopedic Surgery & Pulmonary Embolism (PE)

1. Patrick has a possible pulmonary embolism (PE). What are his significant risk factors for a PE?

2. List three priority nursing diagnoses for pulmonary embolism.

3. Discuss the difference between sub-therapeutic, therapeutic, and prolonged partial thromboplastin time.

4. Due to the recent surgical procedure and hemoglobin of 9.2, would a heparin drip be contraindicated? Why?

5. Reflection is a vital part of the learning process. Discuss what went well during the simulation experience, and what areas need improvement.

6. Chart on the care that you provided Patrick per the educator's guidelines.

Cardiac & Acute Coronary Syndrome (Adult)

Goals/Outcomes of Simulation Exercise

- Students will perform a focused assessment in response to changes in a patient's condition.
- Students will prioritize and initiate nursing interventions upon recognition of abnormal findings.
- Students will evaluate effectiveness of nursing interventions.
- Students will demonstrate effective communication.

Acute Patient Information

It is the day shift (0700) and students will provide care to David Arens, a 65-year-old male who sustained a left mid-shaft femoral fracture yesterday when he fell an estimated 15–20 feet from the roof of his barn. David's admitting hemoglobin was 9.0 g/dL. The fractured femur was stabilized during surgery with screws and a plate. Estimated blood loss during surgery was 300 mL. One unit of packed red blood cells (PRBCs) was transfused in the operating room. Significant ecchymosis is reported in the left thigh. No other significant injuries were sustained during the fall.

David is alert and oriented to person, place, and time. He rested well throughout the night shift and his leg pain has been controlled with the use of a morphine patient-controlled analgesia (PCA). He rated his leg pain at a "1–2" on a scale of 0–5 for the night nurse. At 0600 vital signs were as follows: blood pressure 138/86, apical pulse 84 beats per minute, respirations 18 per minute, tympanic temperature 98.8 °F, and oxygen saturation 96% on room air. The 0600 lab results are as follows: white blood cell count (WBC) 12 μL, hemoglobin (Hgb) 9.2 g/dL, and hematocrit (Hct) 26.1%. His indwelling urinary catheter had 850 mL of clear yellow urine output during the night shift. He has an 18 gauge IV in his right forearm infusing 5% dextrose 0.45% sodium chloride (NaCl) with 20 mEq of potassium chloride (KCl)/liter infusing at 100 mL/hr.

David's lung sounds are clear. He is compliant with his incentive spirometer, using it every hour for five breaths while awake and demonstrating proper usage. He reports mild nausea. David's oral intake during the night consisted of a few ice chips. David's bowel sounds are hypoactive with positive reports of flatus. Equal bilateral pedal pulses are palpated. Slight edema is observed in the left lower leg rated at a 1 +.

David has been awake since 0500. He states that as a farmer, he is "used to getting up early." He expresses concern that he is "stressed" over who will continue to keep his farm up and running while he is in the hospital. He has 60 dairy cows that need to be milked every morning and evening. David informed the night nurse that he does not like to "lay around" and that he rarely watches "the junk on TV." He notes that he may have a hard time with the recovery process. He further stated, "All there is to do is sit and worry about all the things I should be doing." David requested a cigarette multiple times on the night shift. Students will begin care of David at 0730.

Other Relevant Patient Information

- 1/2 pack per day (PPD) smoker since age 25
- Height 5'11"
- Weight 289 pounds

- Previous medical diagnoses include: hypertension, hyperlipidemia, nicotine addiction, and obesity.
- David's younger brother Greg had a myocardial infarction (MI) three months ago and underwent a triple bypass; he reports that his dad "died of heart trouble"; his mother is living and is in good health; he has no siblings other than Greg
- Current medications: lisinopril 20 mg daily, hydrochlorothiazide (HCTZ) 50 mg daily, and Zocor 40 mg every evening.
- No known allergies

Guidelines for Student Preparation

For student success, a review of the following medications and skills are required prior to the simulation exercise. Be sure to review Chapter 1 for further student guidelines. As students review medications the following information should be noted: the trade and generic names, the indications of each medication, safe dosage ranges, primary nursing implications, and common side effects.

- Medications used within this simulation include: lisinopril, hydrochlorothiazide (HCTZ), Zocor, Lovenox, Claforan (IV), aspirin, morphine (IV), nitroglycerin (sublingual), and Lopressor (IV).
- Intravenous (IV) push medications such as morphine and Lopressor are required for this simulation exercise. Administration of medications via IV has special considerations and precautions which should be reviewed prior to the simulation exercise.
- Students should fully review the assessment process. Be aware that a patient chart will be available for review during the simulation exercise.
- Students should be able to demonstrate how to manually obtain all patient vital signs including blood pressure, apical pulse, respirations, oxygen saturation, and temperature.
- Students should review the application of oxygen via various methods.
- Students will need to demonstrate the insertion of a second IV site and the administration of IV fluids. Priming IV tubing setup should be reviewed.
- Students must demonstrate proper assessment technique related to the patient pain and the utilization of a patient-controlled analgesia (PCA).
- Students must demonstrate the proper application of a 5-lead cardiac telemetry monitor. Students should be able to evaluate the rhythm strip produced during the scenario.
- Students should review the process associated with providing a comprehensive verbal report to a healthcare provider and fellow teammates.

- Students must verbalize therapeutic communication.
- Students must be able to understand the following lab values: white blood cell count (WBC), hemoglobin (Hgb), and hematocrit (Hct).
- Students should understand the process involved in obtaining verbal physician's orders via telephone.
- Students must demonstrate proper documentation of medications on the medication administration record (MAR). Students may be required to write a nursing note in relation to the simulation events.

Student Simulation Roles

The student simulation roles are as follows: a supervisor, medication nurse, assessment nurse, and family member. The educator may choose to restructure roles as deemed necessary. For further review of the student roles refer to Chapter 1 of this text. Roles may be assigned prior to the simulation exercise start. It is imperative that students are prepared for all potential roles. Students may consult each other as the simulation exercise progresses. Accuracy needs to be ensured and students may choose to double-check the patient's vital signs and the medications being administered. The educator may reserve the right to grade students on an individual basis, especially if one member of the group is clearly unprepared for the exercise.

Simulation Grade

The educator will provide specific information related to the grading of the simulation exercise. The student's grade will be affected by the timely completion of skills with accuracy. The grading grid presented within this text recommends the following guidelines for grade construction.

1. Beginning Steps: (10%): This includes washing your hands, introducing yourself to the patient, explaining the plan of care, checking the proper patient identification (use two indicators), providing privacy, and donning gloves or applying the appropriate PPE as necessary.
2. Assessment (30%): Prioritize the patient assessment; recall the ABC's (airway, breathing, and circulation). The assessment should remain focused on key patient priorities. The first set of vital signs will be taken manually to ensure that students can accurately obtain an apical pulse, respirations, and blood pressure. Students should demonstrate the usage of all needed equipment. For example, to obtain the patient's oxygen saturation, correctly apply the

device and wait for the educator to verbally provide the reading. As students assess the patient, formulate nursing diagnoses and plan interventions to implement. The primary focus for this simulation exercise is the patient's cardiac status.

3. Report (10%): Students will need to call the primary care provider with report on the patient status. Verbal orders will be given and students should be prepared to take verbal orders via phone. Prior to calling the health care provider, make sure all pertinent patient information is assessed. Organize how you will report patient data to the physician. It is the role of the supervisor to call the health care provider.

4. Implementation (30%): Performance of various nursing skills needs to be done in an accurate and timely manner. See the above information for content to review. Orders will be given for the team to carry out. Be sure to implement the physician's orders in a timely fashion. Students should communicate with other departments (i.e. lab and x-ray) orders which need to be carried out.

5. Evaluation (10%): Evaluate each intervention performed. After students perform an action, they should then question if the action resulted in the desired outcome; if not, formulation of other interventions may be required. Evaluate all medications administered. Re-check the patient's vital signs as this is required.

6. Student Professionalism (10%): Professional dress, proper communication, display of teamwork, preparedness for the scenario, and adaptation to stress will make up the final portion of the simulation grade.

Family Member Information

David was repairing a hail-damaged barn roof when he fell an estimated 15–20 feet. He had been working long hours and was exhausted. David has not been taking good care of himself. He is a "meat and potatoes kind of guy who puts gravy on everything." His primary doctor has encouraged weight loss to reduce his high blood pressure and cholesterol. His younger brother Greg had a triple bypass three months ago. David smokes half a pack of cigarettes per day. He has frequently been asking to go outside to have a cigarette because he claims it will make him feel better. David is a "tough guy" and usually does not complain of pain. The student assigned the role of family member should reassure David that matters relating to his farm are being taken care of. As his condition deteriorates, the student who plays the role of family member should be sure to ask questions about the nursing interventions performed.

Case Study for Simulation 4
Cardiac & Acute Coronary Syndrome

1. David realizes that he might be having a heart attack. He asks you what a heart attack is and how it occurs. You explain that:
2. What patient information could be provided to reduce the risk of a second acute coronary syndrome event?
3. Explain why each medication/intervention is used in the treatment of a MI.
4. How frequently will you monitor David's vital signs? Why?
5. A variety of lab tests were ordered on David. Explain why each lab test was ordered.
6. After Dr. Cooper arrives, he states that ST elevation is observed on the electrocardiogram (EKG). Why is ST elevation a significant finding?
7. List three priority nursing diagnoses for David.
8. Reflection is a vital part of the learning process. Discuss what went well during the simulation experience, and what areas need improvement.
9. Chart on the care that you provided David per the educator's guidelines.

Integument & Wound Care (Adult)

Goals/Outcomes of Simulation Exercise

- Students will prioritize nursing interventions based on assessment of a patient with an integumentary disorder.

- Students will demonstrate skill components related to a central catheter and wound care.

- Students will assess the patient's current emotional state and provide appropriate therapeutic communication.

- Students will provide education regarding home plan of care to patient and family.

Acute Patient Information

It is the day shift (0700) and students will provide care to Shirley Griggs, a 66-year-old female patient who underwent a bowel resection three days ago. A biopsy obtained during a routine colonoscopy tested positive for carcinoma and a bowel resection was recommended. During surgery a segment of the large bowel and several lymph nodes were removed. A small abscess was discovered and the surgical wound was left open. The exact cause of the abscess could not be determined, but the surgeon believes it may have formed as a complication of a ruptured diverticulum. A culture was obtained and Shirley tested positive for methicillin-resistant staphylococcus aureus (MRSA). No fecal diversion (colostomy) was created during the surgery. Shirley has an open midline abdominal incision that measures 9 cm in length by 3 cm in width by 2 cm in depth. Personal protective equipment (PPE) should be used, as contact precautions have been instituted. During the last dressing change the nurse reported the following information: (a) moderate amount of yellow-brown exudate, (b) the wound base was beefy red with granulation, and (c) a slight foul odor. Shirley tolerated the last dressing change without difficulty.

Today is Shirley's postoperative day number three. Shirley is alert and orientated to person, place, and time. The night nurse reports that she rested well and has been using her morphine patient-controlled analgesia (PCA) as needed; 8 mg was self-administered throughout the night (2300–0630). Shirley has reported severe nausea during the past two days and her oral intake has consisted of ice chips. A triple lumen central line was inserted during surgery in the left subclavian. Central line infusions include: (a) dextrose 5% with 0.45% of sodium chloride (NaCl) and 20 mEq of potassium chloride (KCl)/liter at 75 mL/hr in the distal lumen, (b) morphine PCA in the distal lumen with the primary IV fluids, and (c) parenteral nutrition (PN) in the medial lumen. Vancomycin IV is ordered for 0800 and will be infused in the proximal line after ordered labs are drawn (trough).

Shirley's last set of vital signs at 0600 were as follows: respirations 16 per minute at rest; regular apical pulse 76 beats per minute at rest, blood pressure 134/78, tympanic temperature 100.2 °F, and oxygen saturation 97% on room air. The 0600 lab results are as follows: white blood cell count (WBC) 17.4 µL, hemoglobin (Hgb) 10.2 g/dL, and albumin 2.0 g/dL. The night nurse reports that Shirley's lung sounds were clear but diminished in the bases. She has an occasional cough with minimal sputum production. Bowel sounds are hypoactive. Shirley reports flatus. The night nurse reported slight pedal edema. Pedal pulses were present and strong. She voided 250 mL of clear urine with no difficulty at 0530.

The night nurse states that Shirley is very concerned about her diagnosis of cancer and "what the future holds." She becomes teary eyed when she discusses the diagnosis stating, "I know they caught it early but it still really scares me." Shirley has also commented on the fact that she feels so "contaminated" with everyone in gowns and gloves. She states, "I want to see my grandkids." Shirley further relays that she comes from a large family and visiting with them is important. She does not want to "spread germs" to her family. An oncologist will make rounds later this morning to further review prognosis and further treatment recommendations.

Other Relevant Patient Information

- Past medical diagnoses: osteoporosis, hypertension and diverticulitis
- Previous surgeries: hysterectomy at age 54
- Past history of smoking: began smoking at the age of 16, 1 pack per day, quit at age 54 following hysterectomy surgery
- Height 5'3"
- Weight 140 pounds
- Current medications: multivitamin one tablet daily, calcium 600 mg plus vitamin D 200 IU one tablet daily, Hyzaar 50 mg/12.5 mg daily in the morning, and ASA EC 81 mg daily in the morning; all medications listed are via the oral route
- Allergies: no known food or drug allergies

Guidelines for Student Preparation

For student success, a review of the following medications and skills are required prior to the simulation exercise. Be sure to review Chapter 1 for further student guidelines. As students review medications the following information should be noted: the trade and generic names, the indications of each medication, safe dosage ranges, primary nursing implications, and common side effects.

- Medications used within this simulation include: vancomycin IV, morphine PCA, multivitamin, calcium + vitamin D, Hyzaar, and ASA. Primary IV fluid of 5% dextrose with 0.45% of sodium chloride (NaCl) and 20 mEq of potassium chloride (KCl)/liter will be infusing. Parental nutrition (PN) will also be ordered. Students must ensure that the ordered IV fluids are infusing at the correct rates.
- Students should review how to calculate IV medication infusion rates.
- Students should understand guidelines associated with a triple lumen central line. The fluids infusing in the proximal, medial, and distal ports are indicated above.
- A vancomycin trough lab is to be drawn from the central line prior to vancomycin administration. Students should review how to obtain a blood sample from a central line.
- A morphine PCA is ordered. Review the nursing implications related to this method of medication delivery.

- Students should fully review the assessment process. Review the provided patient chart during the simulation exercise.
- Review data relating to instituting contact precautions in a patient with MRSA. Understand how to correctly apply and remove personal protective equipment (PPE).
- Student will be required to demonstrate how to obtain a full set of vital signs.
- Students must educate the patient on proper use of the incentive spirometer.
- Students must demonstrate how to accurately perform a dressing change. Be sure to assess and measure the wound. Pre-medicate the patient prior to the dressing change. Review proper terms/vocabulary which should be used to describe a wound.
- Students must verbalize therapeutic communication. Review the patient information above; pre-plan how you will comfort the patient.
- Fully review the information provided to the family member. Pre-plan how to answer and address the family member's questions and concerns.
- Students should be able to understand how the following lab values affect wound healing: white blood cell count (WBC), hemoglobin (Hgb), and albumin.
- Students should review the process of giving an oral report upon the conclusion of the simulation exercise.
- Students must demonstrate proper documentation of medications on the medication administration record (MAR). Information during the simulation event such as vital signs should be recorded by students for later documentation.

Student Simulation Roles

The student simulation roles are as follows: supervisor, medication nurse, assessment nurse, and family member. The educator may choose to restructure roles as deemed necessary. For further review of the student roles refer to Chapter 1. Roles may be assigned prior to the simulation exercise start. It is imperative that students are prepared for all potential roles. Students may consult each other as the simulation exercise progresses. Accuracy needs to be ensured and students may choose to double-check the patient's vital signs and the medications being administered. The educator may reserve the right to grade students on an individual basis, especially if one member of the team is clearly unprepared for the exercise.

As students prepare for this simulation it is important to note the number of required skills which will need to be completed. A dressing change on a surgical wound, a blood draw from a central line, administration of oral and IV medications, and a thorough patient assessment will need to be performed by the simulation team. The recommended length of time for this simulation is 20–30 minutes. Students must ensure that skills are prepared for and that all team members are actively participating in the exercise.

Simulation Grade

The educator will provide specific information related to the grading of the simulation exercise. The student's grade will be affected by the timely completion of skills with accuracy. The grading grid presented within this text recommends the following guidelines for grade construction.

1. Beginning Steps (10%): This includes washing hands, introducing oneself to the patient, explaining the plan of care, checking the proper patient identification (use two indicators), providing privacy, and donning gloves or applying the appropriate personal protective equipment (PPE) as necessary. Carefully review the PPE guidelines for contact precautions. Understand how to correctly apply PPE and what items should be donned. Skills will need to be performed with PPE donned.

2. Assessment (30%): Prioritize the patient assessment. The assessment should remain focused on key patient priorities. Vital signs will be taken manually to ensure that students can accurately obtain an apical pulse and respirations. Students should demonstrate the usage of all needed equipment. For example, to obtain the patient's oxygen saturation, correctly apply the device and wait for the educator to verbally provide the reading. Wound care is a priority for this simulation exercise. Understand how to measure and assess a wound. Use proper terms and vocabulary when assessing the wound. Students should assess the central line dressing site and ensure that all ordered IV fluids are infusing at the correct rate.

3. Implementation (30%): Performance of various nursing skills needs to be done in an accurate and timely manner. See the above information of content to review. Significant points may be deducted if a medication error is made. Note that a blood sample will need to be obtained from the central catheter prior to the administration of vancomycin. A dressing change on an open abdominal wound will need to be performed. Students should review dressing change technique as taught in laboratory or clinical. Pre-medicate the patient prior to the dressing change to reduce pain. Patient education and review of how to use the incentive sprirometer (IS) should be covered. Provide holistic care and comfort to the patient and demonstrate therapeutic communication.

4. Evaluation (10%): Evaluate each intervention performed. After students perform an action, question if the action resulted in the desired outcome. Evaluation for this simulation may include repeated vital signs, reflection on how the patient tolerated the dressing change, pain, and response to emotional support. Reinforcement of previously taught information is expected.

5. Verbal Report (10%): Upon the conclusion of the simulation exercise students will be required to provide a verbal report to the nurse who will continue patient care. The verbal report should be clear, concise, and organized. Effective communication must be demonstrated.

6. Student Professionalism (10%): Professional dress, proper communication, display of teamwork, preparedness for the scenario, and adaptation to stress will make up the final portion of the simulation grade.

Family Member Information

You arrive to visit your mother today and question the need for gowns and gloves. Is this all really necessary? Do I have to wear a gown and gloves too? I have two small children at home. The discharge nurse spoke with you about changing your mother's dressing daily when she goes home. The physician would like dressing changes done daily and the patient requests a family member do the procedure. You specifically came today to observe the dressing change. You are feeling optimistic today because the surgeon reported the cancer had not spread to any other areas. You are thankful she had the routine colonoscopy.

Case Study for Simulation 5
Integument & Wound Care (Adult)

1. Shirley's colorectal cancer was discovered during a routine colonoscopy. Discuss the recommendations for when a colonoscopy should be performed. What are the associated risk factors of colorectal cancer?

2. A morphine PCA is ordered. Discuss the nursing considerations of a morphine PCA. What side effects should the nurse monitor for?

3. The following lab results were reported: white blood cell count (WBC) 17.4 μL, hemoglobin (Hgb) 10.2 g/dL, and serum albumin 2.0 g/dL. Discuss how these lab results relate to wound healing.

4. Discuss the pathophysiology of wound healing.

5. Red man syndrome can occur with IV vancomycin. Discuss the signs and symptoms of this complication and how to prevent it.

6. List three primary nursing diagnoses for Shirley.

7. Shirley Griggs has a triple lumen central catheter inserted. Discuss guidelines for care of this type of central catheter.

8. Parenteral nutrition (PN) has been ordered. Discuss the nursing considerations of PN administration.

9. Reflection is a vital part of the learning process. Discuss what went well during the simulation experience, and what areas need improvement.

10. Chart on the care that you provided Shirley Griggs per the educator's guidelines.

Brain Attack (formerly called Cerebrovascular Accident [CVA])

Goals/Outcomes of Simulation Exercise

- Students will prioritize an assessment and communicate relevant findings to the primary health care provider.
- Students will demonstrate skill components related to a tracheostomy and gastrostomy tube (G-tube).
- Students will assess the family's response to changes in a patient's condition.
- Students will provide support to a patient and family coping with lifestyle changes.

Acute Patient Information

It is the day shift (0700) and students will provide care to Eva Nelson, an 88-year-old female patient who resides in a long-term care facility. Three months ago, Eva was admitted to the long-term care facility following an ischemic brain attack. Complications from the attack resulted in a tracheostomy and placement of a gastrostomy tube (G-tube). Eva has right-sided hemiplegia and requires assistance with all activities of daily living.

In report the night nurse states that Eva's tracheostomy required suctioning every 3 to 4 hours. The certified nursing assistants (CNAs) noted congestion and weak coughing beginning at 2200. Her vital signs have remained stable. Eva's last set of vital signs at 0500 were as follows: respirations 18 per minute at rest, irregular pulse 94 beats per minute at rest, blood pressure 118/64, tympanic temperature 99.8 °F, and oxygen saturation 96% on room air following tracheal suctioning. She was last suctioned at 0500. A moderate amount of clear sputum was suctioned. The night nurse reports that Eva's oxygen saturations were 90% on room air prior to suctioning. Eva's lung sounds are clear with a few crackles in the bases.

Eva is non-verbal but follows staff movement with her eyes. She nods in agreement occasionally. It is unclear to what extent Eva understands verbal communication. Some nurses have reported that she responds more to loud talking.

Other Relevant Patient Information

- Past medical diagnoses include: hypertension (HTN), high cholesterol, atrial fibrillation, myocardial infarction 5 years ago, depression, and urinary retention
- Previous surgeries: Cholecystectomy, total left hip replacement 10 years ago
- Height 5'6"
- Weight 155 pounds
- Current medications: potassium chloride 20 mEq daily, Lasix 20 mg daily, Colace 100 mg daily, digoxin 0.125 mg daily, Ditropan 5 mg twice daily, metoprolol 50 mg daily, Plavix 75 mg daily, Accupril 20 mg daily, Zocor 10 mg daily, Bactrim 80 mg/400 mg daily, and Zoloft 50 mg daily; all medications are to be administered through the G-tube
- Allergies: sulfa

Guidelines for Student Preparation

For student success, a review of the following medications and skills are required prior to the simulation exercise. Be sure to review Chapter 1 for further student guidelines. As students review medications the following information should be noted: the trade and generic name, the indications of each medication, safe dosage ranges, primary nursing implications, and common side effects.

- ■ Medications used within this simulation include: potassium chloride, Lasix, Colace, digoxin, Ditropan, metoprolol, Plavix, Accupril, Zocor, Bactrim, and Zoloft.
- ■ All medications are to be administered through the gastrostomy tube (G-tube), review the procedure of administering medications via this route.
- ■ Dosage calculations and crushing medications will be required.
- ■ Students should fully review the assessment process. Be aware that a patient chart will be available for review during the simulation exercise.
- ■ Students will be required to demonstrate how to obtain a full set of vital signs on the human patient simulator (HPS).
- ■ Students must demonstrate sterile tracheostomy suctioning and a tracheostomy dressing change.
- ■ Although the patient is non-verbal students should be sure to communicate with the patient and explain the plan of care and procedures being performed.
- ■ Fully review the information provided to the family member. Pre-plan how to address their questions and concerns. Question why the family member may have this response to the nursing care being provided.
- ■ Students should be prepared to notify the primary physician in regards to abnormal assessment findings and understand the process for receiving verbal orders via phone. A blank physician's order sheet will be provided for transcription of orders.
- ■ Students must demonstrate proper documentation of medications on the medication administration record (MAR). Information during the simulation event such as vital signs should be recorded by students for later documentation.

Student Simulation Roles

The student simulation roles are as follows: a supervisor, medication nurse, assessment nurse, and family member (son/daughter). The educator may choose to restructure roles as deemed necessary. For further review of the student roles refer to Chapter 1 of this text. Roles may be assigned just prior to the simulation exercise start. It is imperative that students are prepared for all potential roles. Students may consult each other as the simulation exercise progresses. Students may choose to double-check the patient's vital signs and the medications being administered. The educator may reserve the right to grade students on an individual basis, especially if one member of the team is clearly unprepared for the exercise.

Simulation Grade

The educator will provide specific information related to the grading of the simulation exercise. The student's grade will be affected by the timely completion of skills with accuracy. The grading grid presented within this text recommends the following guidelines for grade construction.

1. **Beginning Steps (10%):** This includes washing hands, introducing oneself to the patient, explaining the plan of care, checking patient identification, providing privacy, and donning gloves or applying the appropriate personal protective equipment (PPE) as necessary.

2. **Assessment (16%):** Prioritize the patient assessment; recall the ABC's (airway, breathing, and circulation). Assessment should remain focused on key patient priorities. Vital signs will be taken manually to ensure that students can accurately obtain an apical pulse and respirations. Students should demonstrate the usage of all equipment.

3. **Implementation (44%):** Performance of various nursing skills needs to be done in an accurate and timely manner. See the above information for content to review. Tracheostomy suctioning will be required and the tracheostomy dressing will be changed. Students should review sterile technique. Medications will be administered through a gastrostomy tube. Significant points may be deducted for medication errors. Students should pre-plan communication with the family member.

4. **Evaluation (10%):** Evaluate each intervention performed. After students perform an intervention they should question if the action resulted in the desired outcome. Evaluation for this simulation may include repeated vital signs, recheck of the oxygen saturation, evaluation of lung sounds, and further communication with the family member.

5. **Verbal Report (10%):** Students will be required to notify the primary physician in regards to abnormal assessment findings in patient condition. The verbal report should be clear, concise, and organized. All pertinent patient information should be included in the report. Effective communication must be demonstrated. Verbal orders will be obtained.

6. **Student Professionalism (10%):** Professional dress, proper communication, display of teamwork, preparedness for the scenario, and adaptation to stress will make up the final portion of the simulation grade.

Family Member Information

You arrive today and your mother sounds congested. You would like an explanation for this. What is being done about this new symptom? Does the physician know? Should your mother be admitted to the hospital? Ask the nurses caring for your mother about their level of experience. Have they suctioned a tracheostomy before? Question each medication administered. You feel that you need to be your mother's voice because she is unable to speak. Speech therapy was unsuccessful in assisting your mother use any devices to help her communicate.

Case Study for Simulation 6 Brain Attack (formerly called Cerebrovascular Accident [CVA])

1. Discuss the pathophysiology of artery blockage from plaque in an ischemic stroke. There are two types of ischemic strokes: thrombotic and embolic.
2. List three priority nursing diagnoses for Eva in regard to her deteriorating respiratory status.
3. Multiple medications are administered via a gastrostomy tube (G-tube) in this simulation exercise. One complication that may arise is a plugged or blocked G-tube. Discuss how the nurse should prevent the G-tube from clogging.
4. Discuss what actions could be used to assist Eva with communication.
5. Eva has an increased risk of aspiration. List the factors that increase her aspiration risk and identify ways in which the nurse can decrease aspiration risk.
6. Reflection is a vital part of the learning process. Discuss what went well during the simulation experience, and what areas need improvement.
7. Chart on the care that you provided Eva Nelson per the educator's guidelines.

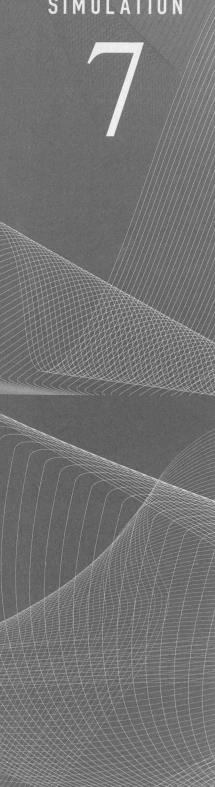

SIMULATION

7

Cancer & End of Life (Adult)

Goals/Outcomes of Simulation Exercise

- Students will prioritize nursing interventions based on assessment of the patient with cancer.
- Students will apply principles of asepsis for a neutropenic patient's protection.
- Students will demonstrate skill components of advanced intravenous therapy for an implanted port.
- Students will verbalize effective communication to members of the health care team.
- Students will discuss nursing interventions related to end of life care.

Acute Patient Information

It is the evening shift (1500) and students will provide care to Jean Hafner, a 55-year-old female patient with stage IV pancreatic cancer. She was a pack-a-day smoker for over 35 years and quit smoking when cancer was discovered 5 months ago. Jean underwent a laparoscopic Whipple procedure. She has had a slow recovery from the surgery and a jejunostomy tube was inserted for feedings. Treatments of chemotherapy with gemcitabine were given after her recovery from Whipple surgery. Jean has an implanted port in her left upper chest for chemotherapy. She has been receiving parenteral nutrition at night due to her jejunostomy tube functioning improperly. She is hospitalized to have the jejunostomy tube removed and for pain control. On admission she had severe abdominal pain, a fever, and a history of a low neutrophil count three days ago. Reverse isolation precautions have been instituted.

Jean is quiet and is confused at times. She knows who she is but has no idea why she is hospitalized or what the year is. She was admitted directly from her home after the home care nurse saw her this morning and phoned her oncologist for admitting orders. She is just getting settled in her room now by the certified nursing assistant while you are getting a report from the admitting nurse. He reports that Jean is alert but has periods of confusion. Her skin is hot to touch and she is too weak to ambulate. Jean voided a small amount of dark amber urine on admission. Her vitals were as follows: blood pressure 92/58, apical pulse 48 beats per minute, respirations 22 breaths per minute, tympanic temperature 101.4 °F, and oxygen saturation 83% on room air. She has an implanted port in the left chest area that has not been accessed. She has decreased breath sounds bilaterally, with an occasional weak dry cough. Jean's abdomen is slightly distended with no bowel sounds. The admitting nurse has inserted a nasogastric tube (NG) per physician's orders. Jean rates her pain at a 5 of 5. She states, "The pain is mostly in my stomach but I hurt all over." The admitting nurse also tells you that Jean is talking about dying and her wish is to die at home.

There are no lab results for Jean at this time but you are told by family that her white counts "were very low three days ago." Clinic records confirm the low WBC. Labs will be drawn from the implanted port when it is accessed. Jean has a fentanyl drip ordered along with primary IV fluids.

The admission nurse states that Jean came in with one family member, who is very concerned about her. He says the family member seems to understand how sick Jean is. Jean lives alone 30 miles from town. Various family members feel 30 miles is too far for them to continue driving daily to care for her at home. Plans for Jean to be admitted to the hospice unit in town are in progress. Jean does not want to leave her home and repeatedly tells the family she wishes to die at home. Family members have been arguing in the process of making end of life decisions.

4. Evaluation (10%): Evaluate each intervention performed. After students perform an intervention they should question if the action resulted in the desired outcome; if not, formulation of other interventions may be required. Evaluate all medications administered. Re-check the patient's vital signs as this is required.
5. Postmortem Care (10%): Postmortem care will need to be discussed.
6. Student Professionalism (10%): Professional dress, proper communication, display of teamwork, preparedness for the scenario, and adaptation to stress will make up the final portion of the simulation grade.

Family Member Information

You came to the hospital with your mother and are upset with the rest of your family. They think that your mother should be moved to a hospice unit in town. You think she should die at home as she is requesting. You are the only sibling who feels this way. Your mother is a widow and has shared with you that she wants to die soon and be with your late father. She has a strong faith and feels it is time to go "home." There has been a great deal of arguing with your siblings about your mother and you are very tired of the drama. You have notified her priest to let him know how sick your mother is. You are tearful but remain close to your mother. The remainder of your family has been notified that she has been admitted to the hospital.

Case Study for Simulation 7
Cancer & End of Life (Adult)

1. Discuss neutropenic significance in this scenario.
2. Define symptoms of distress at the end of life.
3. Discuss goals for end of life care.
4. Describe postmortem cares.
5. What are the signs and symptoms of the dying process?
6. The topic of death may be difficult. Discuss methods of coping used by the professional nurse in the event of a patient's death.
7. Chart on the end of life cares that you provided Jean Hafner per the educator's guidelines.

Assessment & Medication Administration (Pediatric)

Goals/Outcomes of Simulation Exercise

- Students will demonstrate an age-appropriate assessment and identify abnormal findings.
- Students will prioritize nursing interventions based on assessment.
- Students will demonstrate skill components of intravenous initiation and medication administration.
- Students will verbalize age-appropriate communication techniques.

Acute Patient Information

It is the day shift (0900) and students will provide care to Scotty Bauer, a 6-month-old male infant diagnosed with bacterial pneumonia and dehydration early this morning. A clinic nurse has just escorted Scotty and his grandparent to the pediatric unit for admission. Scotty's grandparent states that he was diagnosed with pneumonia 3 days ago and was prescribed Zithromax. The grandparent states, "He is getting worse rather than better." Over the course of the last 12 hours the grandparent reports that Scotty has had increased difficulty breathing stating, "It was really fast." Scotty's liquid intake has decreased by 75% and he refuses to eat any solid foods. His grandparent reports that he had two wet diapers in the last 12 hours and several episodes of diarrhea. The grandparent observed that his buttocks are very red and look "like a yeast rash similar to one he had 2 months ago."

The clinic nurse reports that Scotty makes eye contact but does not appear interested in his surroundings. His respirations at the clinic were 62 breaths per minute, and his oxygen saturation was 88% on room air. After ½ liter of oxygen was applied his saturations increased to 93% (he arrived to the unit with portable oxygen). The clinic nurse observed a harsh productive cough, bilateral course crackles, intercostal retractions, use of accessory muscles, nasal flaring, and his clothing smelled of cigarette smoke. Scotty's skin was pale, his capillary refill was 3 seconds, no tearing was observed with crying, and his mucous membranes were dry. The clinic nurse auscultated a heart murmur. An innocent heart murmur was previously noted in his clinic chart. Scotty refused a bottle despite multiple attempts by his grandparent. Scotty's grandparent has been very attentive. His mother could not be reached for admission consent.

A chest x-ray showed consolidation in the bilateral lower lobes; greater on the right. Influenza and respiratory syncytial virus (RSV) tests were negative. Complete blood count (CBC) and chemistry panels (electrolytes) are pending.

Other Relevant Patient Information

- Past medical diagnosis: otitis media, 2 months ago
- Prenatal history: five prenatal visits (all during the last trimester)
- Born at 38 weeks; weight 6 pounds 2 ounces
- Current weight 15.5 pounds
- Current length 25 inches
- Up to date on immunizations
- Current medications: Zithromax, dose administered today at 0600 (prescription for five doses); the grandparent is unsure if the prescribed dose was administered by the patient's mother yesterday
- Allergies: no known food or drug allergies

Guidelines for Student Preparation

Prior to the simulation exercise students should review the following medication list and prepare to perform the indicated skills. Be sure to read Chapter 1 of the student text for additional guidelines. As students review medications the following information should be noted: the trade and generic names, the indications of each medication, safe dosage ranges, various routes of administration, primary nursing implications, and common side effects.

■ Medications used within the simulation include: cefuroxime (IV), acetaminophen, ibuprofen, Xopenex nebulizer, and IV maintenance fluid of 0.9% sodium chloride (NaCl). An IV fluid bolus of NaCl (one time) will also be ordered. Review how to administer an IV fluid bolus.

■ Review dosage calculations prior to the simulation exercise as calculation will be required during medication administration. Understand how to calculate weight-based medication dosages for pediatrics.

■ Review infant IV access, the proper location (anatomical landmarks), IV cannula size, and safe IV bag volume.

■ Students must be aware of IV considerations related to an infant (i.e. safe rates, monitoring the IV site, and how to properly secure the accessed site).

■ Students should be familiar with the procedure of administering a nebulizer treatment to a 6-month-old infant.

■ Students should fully review the assessment process. Be aware that a patient chart will be available for review during the simulation exercise.

■ Students should demonstrate how to manually obtain all patient vital signs including apical pulse, respirations, oxygen saturation, and temperature. Note that the simulated patient will be an infant. Know the normal range of infant vital signs. Understand the HPS functions to increase competency of these skills.

■ Students should understand how to assess an infant for signs and symptoms of respiratory distress. Human patient simulators may not be able to display signs such as nasal flaring and retractions. Students **MUST** be sure to verbalize when observing for signs of respiratory distress and be specific in order to gain patient data. For example, a student could state, "I am observing for nasal flaring and use of accessory muscles." The educator will then provide information in regards to the assessed data. Points may be deducted if omission of respiratory data occurs.

■ Students should review how to properly apply oxygen to an infant patient.

■ Students should review the process of giving a verbal report to the oncoming shift at the conclusion of the simulation exercise.

■ Talk to the simulator as you would a "real" patient. Be sure to provide age-appropriate care. Ask the grandparent questions as the educator will provide some of the verbal responses (some responses will be provided by the "grandparent"). Consider your approach to a 6-month-old and how you might alter care. Review of age-specific growth and development is recommended.

■ Explain the plan of care to the grandparent. Provide education in regard to medications and procedures. This will be especially important when the IV is started.

■ Reflect on the psychosocial aspects provided in the patient history.

■ Students must demonstrate proper documentation of medications on the medication administration record (MAR). Students may be required to write a nursing note in relation to the simulation events. Information (i.e. vital signs) during the simulation event should be recorded.

Student Simulation Roles

The student simulation roles are as follows: supervisor, medication nurse, assessment nurse, and family member. The educator may choose to restructure roles as deemed necessary. For further review of the student roles refer to Chapter 1 of the student text. Roles may be assigned just prior to the simulation exercise start. It is imperative that students are prepared for all potential roles. As this is a team effort students may consult each other as the simulation exercise progresses. Accuracy needs to be ensured and students may choose to double-check the patient's vital signs and the medications being administered. The educator may reserve the right to grade students on an individual basis, especially if one member of the team is clearly unprepared for the exercise.

Simulation Grade

The educator will provide specific information related to the grading of the simulation exercise. The student's grade will be affected by the timely completion of skills with accuracy. The grading grid presented within this text recommends the following guidelines for grade construction.

1. Beginning Steps (10%): This includes washing your hands, introducing yourself to the patient and the caregiver, explaining the plan of care, checking the proper patient identification (use two indicators), providing privacy, and donning gloves or applying the appropriate PPE as necessary.

2. Assessment (30%): Prioritize the assessment; recall the ABC's (airway, breathing, and circulation). The assessment should remain focused on key patient priorities. Vital signs will be taken manually to ensure that students can accurately obtain an apical pulse and respirations. Students should demonstrate the usage of all needed equipment. For example, to obtain the patient's oxygen saturation, correctly apply the device and wait for the educator to verbally provide the reading. Students should further expand upon the patient information learned in report; subjective and objective data should assessed.

3. Implementation (30%): Performance of various nursing skills needs to be done in an accurate and timely manner. See the above information for content to review. Students will be required to administer some of the medications listed above. Calculation of medications doses based upon weight will be required. Significant points may be deducted for medication errors. Be sure to consider all aspects of pediatric medication administration.

4. Evaluation (10%): Evaluate each intervention performed. After students perform an action, question if the action resulted in the desired outcome. Evaluate the medications administered to determine if the desired effect of the medication occurred.

5. Verbal Report (10%): During the simulation exercise students will be required to provide a verbal report. The verbal report should be clear, concise, and organized. Effective communication must be demonstrated.

6. Student Professionalism (10%): Professional dress, proper communication, display of teamwork preparedness for the scenario, and adaptation to stress will make up the final portion of the simulation grade.

Family Member Information

As Scotty's grandparent you are the primary care giver. Your daughter (Scotty's mother), is rarely around and likes to party. When she does provide care for Scotty you suspect that he does not receive good care. He frequently arrives at your house smelling like cigarette smoke, is dirty, and usually has a diaper that has not been changed recently. You worry about your daughter's ability to care for Scotty and are unsure if he got his second dose of Zithromax because he was under your daughter's care when it was scheduled to be given. Your daughter dropped Scotty off at your place yesterday and cannot be reached today to be informed that Scotty has been hospitalized. At this point you are unsure if she would truly care. She has a habit of disappearing for days.

Your daughter delayed telling you about the pregnancy until late because she continued to smoke and drink alcohol during the majority of her pregnancy. Visits to a health care provider did not occur until late in the pregnancy and only after much encouragement on your part. There is currently a question of who Scotty's father is. Though you love your daughter you do not support her lifestyle. You fear for Scotty's welfare and are considering taking legal action to become his primary caregiver.

Case Study for Simulation 8
Assessment & Medication Administration (Pediatric)

1. Scotty is diagnosed with bacterial pneumonia. Viral pneumonia is common in infants. Discuss the differences between bacterial and viral pneumonia.

2. Discuss the signs and symptoms of respiratory decline in infants.

3. Discuss the safety precautions that the nurse must consider when caring for a pediatric patient receiving IV therapy.

4. Discuss appropriate locations that the nurse should consider when selecting an IV site for an infant.

5. What are the primary indications for cefuroxime? What is the dosage range of cefuroxime for infants (i.e. mg/kg)? What are common side effects that must be monitored for?

6. A red rash was observed by Scotty's grandparent and the admission nurse. A yeast rash is suspected. Discuss the risk factors for a yeast infection.

7. Multiple nursing interventions were performed to improve Scotty's condition. What assessment data will determine if Scotty's condition is improving?

8. Several concerns relating to Scotty's social history arise during this simulation. What pieces of data are concerning? What is the RN's role in addressing these concerns?

9. Reflection is a vital part of the learning process. Discuss what went well during the simulation experience, and what areas need improvement.

10. Chart on the care that you provided Scotty per the educator's guidelines.

Respiratory & Croup (Infant)

Goals/Outcomes of Simulation Exercise

- Students will demonstrate age-appropriate assessment and identify abnormal findings.
- Students will prioritize emergent interventions.
- Students will transcribe and implement verbal physician's orders.
- Student will use therapeutic communication techniques with the patient and family.

Acute Patient Information

It is the evening shift (2100) and students will provide care to Dylan Derheim, a 9-month-old male infant who presents to the emergency department (ED) carried by his parent. As Dylan's parent carries him into the ED you hear loud inspiratory and expiratory stridor. Dylan's parent appears panicked. You immediately bring them back to a treatment room calling for help from your fellow co-workers as you pass by the nurses' station. Dylan's parent reports that he awoke 45 minutes ago with a "barking cough and was gasping for air." No previous assessment data will be provided to students because this patient is just arriving to the ED. Within this simulation exercise students will need to gather all assessment data directly from the HPS and family member. Dr. Giske, the ED physician, is in the department.

Other Relevant Patient Information

- Past medical diagnoses healthy, parent reports a "few colds"
- Prenatal history: mother attended all recommended physician visits, uncomplicated pregnancy
- Born at 39 weeks; weight 7 pounds 8 ounces
- Parent unsure of current weight
- Up to date on immunizations
- Current medications: none
- Breastfed; foods slowly being introduced
- Allergies: no known food or drug allergies

Guidelines for Student Preparation

For student success, a review of the following medications and skills are required prior to the simulation exercise. Be sure to review Chapter 1 for further student guidelines. As students review medications the following information should be noted: the trade and generic names, the indications of each medication, the safe dosage ranges, primary nursing implications, and common side effects.

- Medications used within this simulation include: racemic epinephrine nebulizer, dexamethasone intramuscular (IM), and acetaminophen by mouth.
- Students should review how to calculate medications based upon weight.
- Students should fully review the assessment process. Understand what data might be normal or abnormal in an infant patient.
- Students should understand how to assess an infant for signs and symptoms of respiratory distress. Human patient simulators may not be able to display signs such as nasal flaring and retractions. However,

it is imperative that the nurse monitor for such data. Students **MUST** be sure to state when observing for signs of respiratory distress; be specific in order to gain patient data. For example, a student could state, "I am observing for nasal flaring and use of accessory muscles." The instructor will then provide information in regard to the assessed data. Points may be deducted if omission of respiratory data occurs.

- Students should understand various methods of oxygen application for a 9-month-old.
- Students should understand how to administer a nebulizer treatment to an infant.
- Student will be required to demonstrate how to obtain a full set of vital signs. Know normal vital sign parameters for a 9-month-old.
- Students will be required to verbally state how to obtain a weight on an infant patient.
- Students must understand the procedure of administering an intramuscular (IM) injection to an infant. Understand the proper landmarks and safety considerations.
- Students should understand the process of initiating intravenous (IV) therapy in an infant patient. Review what supplies will be needed.
- Students must demonstrate therapeutic communication with the parent. Review the patient information above and pre-plan how you will comfort the parent in this situation. If a parent is very nervous this may increase the stress level of the infant.
- Educate the parent about the medical condition and interventions being performed.
- Student will need to understand the process of following verbal orders.
- Students will be required to communicate with other departments (i.e., lab and x-ray).
- Students must demonstrate proper documentation of verbal orders and medications administered on the medication administration record (MAR). Information during the simulation event such as vital signs should be recorded by students for later documentation.
- Students should review the process of giving a verbal report to the admission nurse upon the conclusion of the simulation scenario.

Student Simulation Roles

The student simulation roles are as follows: supervisor, medication nurse, assessment nurse, and family member. The educator may choose to restructure roles as deemed necessary. For further review of the student roles refer to Chapter 1 of the student text. Roles will be assigned just prior to the simulation exercise start. It is imperative that students are prepared for all potential roles. Students may consult each other as the simulation exercise progresses. Accuracy needs to be ensured and students may choose to double-check the patient's vital signs and the medications being administered. The educator may reserve the right to grade students on an individual basis, especially if one member of the team is clearly unprepared for the exercise.

Simulation Grade

The educator will provide specific information related to the grading of the simulation exercise. The student's grade will be affected by the timely completion of skills with accuracy. The grading grid presented within this text recommends the following guidelines for grade construction.

1. Beginning Steps (5%): This includes hand hygiene and introducing yourself to the parent. The beginning steps should be brief and students should rapidly begin the patient assessment.
2. Assessment (30%): Prioritize the patient assessment. The assessment should remain focused on key patient priorities. Vital signs will be taken manually to ensure that students can accurately obtain an apical pulse and respirations. Students should demonstrate the usage of all needed equipment. For example, to obtain the patient's oxygen saturation, correctly apply the device and wait for the educator to verbally provide the reading. Respiratory status is the key focus of this simulation scenario. Students should preplan how to focus on a respiratory assessment. Communication of any abnormal findings should occur in a timely fashion. Recall that an emergency department (ED) physician is readily available.
3. Obtained Orders (10%): Students will be given verbal orders from the ED physician. Implementation of verbal orders should occur in a timely manner. Students should clearly communicate all assessment findings with the physician.
4. Implementation (30%): Performance of nursing skills needs to be done in an accurate and timely manner. See the above information for content to review. Significant points may be deducted if a medication error is made. Students will need to administer a nebulizer, oral medications, and an IM medication. Communication with other departments will need to occur. As you implement interventions, remember to provide age-appropriate care. Educate the parent on the plan of care.
5. Evaluation (10%): Evaluate each intervention performed. After students perform an action, question if the action resulted in

the desired outcome. Evaluation for this simulation may include repeated vital signs and re-evaluation of any abnormal findings from the first assessment.

6. **Admission (5%):** Upon the conclusion of the simulation exercise students will be required to provide a verbal report to the nurse who will admit this patient to the acute care facility. The verbal report should be clear, concise, and organized. Effective communication must be demonstrated.

7. **Student Professionalism (10%):** Professional dress, proper communication, display of teamwork, preparedness for the scenario, and adaptation to stress will make up the final portion of the simulation grade.

Family Member Information

Note to student assigned the family role: This is an extremely anxious time for you. Insist on touching, kissing, and providing comfort to your child.

You arrive at the emergency department (ED) with your son Dylan. He awoke 45 minutes ago with a harsh barking cough and couldn't breathe normally. Immediately you knew something was wrong so you brought him to the ED. Dylan did seem to get slightly better in the car (as he was exposed to the cool air outside), but this was only temporary. Dylan is typically healthy and is cared for at home. Dylan has been fussy and has not been nursing well today. He refused to nurse at bedtime. He has had a runny nose and has not been able to sleep well for two days. You have a 4-year-old son at home named Tyler and wonder if he will get sick too.

Ask the nurses many questions. Direct your questions towards the nursing staff as Dr. Giske is "not in the mood" to answer many questions.

Case Study for Simulation 9
Respiratory & Croup (Infant)

1. Dylan is diagnosed with croup. Dylan's parent does not know what croup is. How would you describe this condition?
2. What are the key points of assessment in croup?
3. When reviewing the lab results presented earlier in this chapter, a high lymphocyte and low neutrophil count are observed. What might this indicate? Why might this be important information in the treatment of this patient?
4. List three primary nursing diagnoses for Dylan.
5. Outline a teaching plan for acetaminophen administration.
6. The parent questioned if this condition will affect Dylan's 4-year-old sibling Tyler. How might the nurses respond to this question?
7. Reflection is a vital part of the learning process. Discuss what went well during the simulation experience, and what areas need improvement.
8. Chart on the care you provided Dylan Derheim per the educator's guidelines.

Endocrine & Diabetes (Pediatric)

Goals/Outcomes of Simulation Exercise

- Students will demonstrate an age-appropriate assessment and prioritize nursing interventions.
- Students will calculate an insulin dose based on carbohydrate consumption.
- Students will evaluate and report changes in patient condition.
- Students will instruct a diabetic patient in insulin administration and carbohydrate counting.
- Students will allow the patient to express concerns and fear in regard to diabetic diagnosis.

Acute Patient Information

It is the day shift (0700) and students will provide care to Sarah Holt, a 12-year-old female patient who was transferred to the medical unit from the intensive care unit yesterday with a primary diagnosis of diabetic ketoacidosis. Sarah presented to the emergency department (ED) two days ago after her family found her unresponsive. History per the ED note includes polydipsia, polyuria, and weight loss. Lab urinalysis revealed a urinary tract infection (UTI). The family reports Sarah had flu-like symptoms including nausea, vomiting, and abdominal pain two days prior to admission.

Sarah is somnolent and oriented to person, place, and time. The night nurse reports that she has not been talking much and does not make eye contact with the nursing staff. Sarah has been arguing with her parent and is uncooperative. Her last set of vital signs at 0600 was 22 respirations per minute, apical pulse regular at 72 beats per minute, blood pressure 98/64, tympanic temperature 98.9 °F, and oxygen saturation 99% on room air.

Her initial admission labs were blood glucose 650 mg/dL, serum potassium (K+) 4.8 mEq/L, white blood cell count (WBC) 12.2 μ/L, serum pH 7.20, serum HCO_3 12 mEq/L, BUN 22 mEq/L, urine ketones were positive, and urine tested positive for white and red cells. Lab results at 0600 were blood glucose 84 mg/dL, K+ 3.4 mEq/L, serum pH 7.39, serum HCO_3 15.2 mEq/L, BUN 18, and urine ketones were negative.

Sarah's skin is warm, dry, and pale. Weight is 172 this morning. Lungs are clear and heart tones are normal. Capillary refill time is 3 seconds. A 20 gauge IV is patent in her left forearm with lactated ringers (LR) infusing at 50 mL/hr. The night nurse reports Sarah's urine is clear amber, and her last void was 250 mL at 0500.

Sarah lives with her parent and two younger brothers. She has been involved in music at school but has avoided any sport activities. Her parent says she spends "too much time" in front of the computer and TV and does not spend much time with friends. She is withdrawn from family activities. Her father and mother divorced three years ago, and she does not see her other parent more than once or twice a year.

Other Relevant Patient Information

- Admission diagnosis: diabetic ketoacidosis with new diagnosis of type 1 diabetes, UTI, depression
- Past history of polydipsia, polyuria
- Height 4'8"
- Admission weight 174 pounds
- Current medications: none
- Allergies: none

Guidelines for Student Preparation

Prior to the simulation exercise students should review the following medication list and prepare to perform the indicated skills. Be sure to read Chapter 1 of the student text for additional guidelines. As students review medications the following information should be noted: the trade and generic names, the indications of each medication, safe dosage ranges, various routes of administration, primary nursing implications, and common side effects.

- Medications used within simulation seven include: Lantus and Humalog insulin, Zoloft, Bactrim/Sulfa, IV infusion of sodium chloride (NaCl), saline lock flush, Zofran (oral disintegrating tablet), and 50% dextrose IV push.
- Students will need to understand carbohydrate calculation and corresponding insulin dosage. The breakfast tray will consist of: two pieces of wheat toast, 1/2 banana, one carton of skim milk, and sugar-free jam.
- Students should fully review the assessment process. Be aware that a patient chart will be available for review during the simulation exercise.
- Students should assess the IV site and fluids infusing.
- Students should be able to demonstrate how to manually obtain all patient vital signs including blood pressure, apical pulse, respirations, oxygen saturation, and temperature.
- Students must verbalize therapeutic communication.
- Students should educate the patient on the medications administered during the simulation exercise.
- Students should be familiar with the procedure of flushing a saline lock (SL).
- Students should be prepared to respond to a hypoglycemic reaction.
- Students must demonstrate obtaining a capillary blood glucose reading.
- Students must be able to understand the following lab values: blood glucose, electrolyte panel, CBC, arterial blood gases, and urine ketones.
- Students must demonstrate proper documentation of medications on the medication administration record (MAR). Students may be required to document simulation events at the discretion of the educator. Information during the simulation event should be recorded.
- Students should be prepared to notify the primary health care provider in regard to patient condition and understand the process for receiving verbal orders via phone.

Student Simulation Roles

The student simulation roles are as follows: supervisor, medication nurse, assessment nurse, and family member. The educator may choose to restructure roles as deemed necessary. For further review of the student roles refer to Chapter 1 of the student text. Roles may be assigned prior to the simulation exercise start. It is imperative that students are prepared for all potential roles. Students may consult each other as the simulation exercise progresses. Accuracy needs to be ensured and students may choose to double-check the patient's vital signs and the medications being administered.

Student must recall pediatric guidelines for medication administration. The educator may reserve the right to grade students on an individual basis, especially if one member of the team is clearly unprepared for the exercise.

Simulation Grade

The educator will provide specific information related to the grading of the simulation exercise. The student's grade will be affected by the timely completion of skills with accuracy. The grading grid presented within this text recommends the following guidelines for grade construction.

1. Beginning Steps (10%): This includes washing your hands, introducing yourself to the patient, explaining the plan of care, checking the proper patient identification (use two indicators), providing privacy, and donning gloves or applying the appropriate PPE as necessary (i.e., when checking capillary blood glucose).
2. Assessment (30%): Prioritize the assessment; recall the ABC's (airway, breathing, and circulation). The assessment should remain focused on key priorities in regard to the diabetic patient. The first set of vital signs will be taken manually to ensure that students can accurately obtain an apical pulse, respirations, and blood pressure. Students should demonstrate the usage of all needed equipment. Calculation of carbohydrate intake is necessary for insulin dosage. Students should be sure to assess the patient's psychosocial status.
3. Implementation *Part A* (22%): Performance of various nursing skills needs to be done in an accurate and timely manner. See the above information of content to review. Within this section students will be required to administer some of the medications listed above. Significant points may be deducted for medication errors.

Students must demonstrate the administration of short and long acting insulin. Patient education should occur with medication administration.

4. **Evaluation (10%):** Evaluate each intervention performed. After students perform an action, question if the action resulted in the desired outcome. Evaluate the medications administered to determine if the desired effect of the medication occurred. This may include rechecking the patient's capillary blood glucose.

5. **Verbal Report (10%):** During the simulation exercise, students will be required to provide a verbal report to the primary physician and address all of the concerns that arise during the simulation exercise. The verbal report should be clear, concise, and organized. Effective communication must be demonstrated. Students should understand the process for receiving verbal orders.

6. **Implementation** *Part B* **(8%):** Students must carry out the physician's orders obtained within the verbal report in a timely manner. To ensure all orders are completed, the assessment nurse and supervisor may assist the medication nurse.

7. **Student Professionalism (10%):** Professional dress, proper communication, display of teamwork, preparedness for the scenario, and adaptation to stress will make up the final portion of the simulation grade.

Family Member Information

Sarah has been more withdrawn at home and is spending additional time in her room. Her parent states that she does not find pleasure in activities which she normally enjoys. Her behavior has changed drastically in the past two months. Fighting between Sarah and her brothers has escalated in the past two weeks. Her change in behavior has been difficult for the family. Her parent describes her as depressed and tearful. Sarah's parent further states concern that her school grades have dropped during the past month.

Case Study for Simulation 10
Endocrine & Diabetic (Pediatric)

1. Diabetic ketoacidosis is a potentially life-threatening complication of type 1 diabetes. More serious is hyperglycemic-hyperosmolar nonketotic syndrome. In a comparison table, outline the primary differences between these two life-threatening conditions.

2. Sarah presents with the initial diagnosis of diabetic ketoacidosis. Which findings in her history, lab report, and exam support this diagnosis?

3. What is the expected action the student will take to prevent a hypoglycemic reaction?

4. With the noted psychosocial history for Sarah, what is the priority nursing diagnosis for her behavior in relation to her newly diagnosed diabetes?

5. Discuss information that should be included in a teaching plan for Sarah prior to discharge.

6. Reflection is a vital part of the learning process. Discuss what went well during the simulation experience, and what areas need improvement.

7. Chart on the care that you provided Sarah per the educator's guidelines.

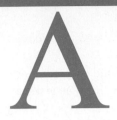

References

Arundell, F., & Cioffi, J. (2005). Using a simulation strategy: An educator's experience. *Nurse Education in Practice*, 5, 296–301.

Brannan J.D., White, A., & Bezanson, J.L. (2008). Simulator effects on cognitive skills and confidence levels. *Journal of Nursing Education*, 47(11), 495–500.

Brimble, M. (2008). Skills assessment using video analysis in a simulated environment: An evaluation. *Paediatric Nursing*, 20(7), 296–301.

Childs, J.C., & Sepples, S. (2006). Clinical teaching by simulation: Lessons learned from a complex patient care scenario. *Nursing Education Perspectives*, 27(3).

Cioffi, J. (2001). Clinical simulations: Development and validation. *Nurse Education Today*, 21, 477–486.

Curtin, M.M., & Dupuis, M.D. (2008). Development of human patient simulations programs: Achieving big results with a small budget. *Journal of Nursing Education*, 47(11), 522–523.

Daniels, R., Nosek, L., & Nicoll, L. (2007). *Contemporary medical–surgical nursing*. Clifton Park, NY: Delmar Cengage Learning.

Daniels, R. (2010). *Delmar's manual of laboratory and diagnostic tests*. (2nd ed.). Clifton Park, NY: Delmar Cengage Learning.

Decker, S., Sportsman, S., Puetz, L., & Billings, L. (2008). The evolution of simulation and its contribution to competency. *The Journal of Continuing Education in Nursing*, 39(2).

Del Bueno, D.J. (2001). Buyer beware: The cost of competence. *Nursing Economics*, 19(6), 250–257.

Feingold, C.E., Calaluce, M., & Kallen, M.A. (2004). Computerized patient model and simulated clinical experiences: Evaluation with baccalaureate nursing students. *Journal of Nursing Education*, 43(4), 156–163.

Goldenberg, D., Andrusyszyn, M.A., & Iwasiw, C. (2005). The effect of classroom simulation on nursing students: Self-efficacy related to health teaching. *Journal of Nursing Education*, 44(7), 310–314.

Harlow, K.C., & Sportsman, S. (2007). An economic analysis of patient simulations for clinical training in nursing education. *Nursing Economics*, 25(1), 24–29.

Hawkins, K., Todd, M., & Manz, J. (2008). A unique simulation teaching method. *Journal of Nursing Education*, 47(11).

Henning, J.M., Lesperance, M., & Harris, J.D. (2007). Developing computer simulations for student assessment. *Athletic Therapy Today*, 12(3), 23–26.

Hertel, J.P., & Millis, G.J. (2002). *Using simulations to promote learning in higher education: An introduction.* Sterling, VA: Stylus.

Janes, B., & Cooper, J. (1996). Simulations in nursing education. *Australian Journal of Advanced Nursing,* 13(4).

Jeffries, P.R. (2005). A framework for designing, implementing, and evaluating simulations used as teaching strategies in nursing. *Nursing Education Perspectives,* 26(2), 96–103.

Jeffries, P.R., & Rizzolo, M.A. (2006). *Summary report. Project title: Designing and implementing models for the innovative use of simulation to teach nursing care of ill adults and children: A national, multi-site, multi-method study.* Retrieved April 11, 2008, from the National League of Nursing Web site: http://www.nln.org/research/LaerdalReport.pdf.

Johnson, J.H., Zerwic, J.J., & Theis, S.L. (1999). Clinical simulation laboratory: An adjunct to clinical teaching. *Nurse Educator,* 24(5), 37–41.

Larew, C., Lessans, S., Spunt, D., Foster, D., & Covington, B. (2004). Innovations in clinical simulation: Application of Brenner's theory in an interactive patient care simulation. *Nursing Education Perspectives,* 27(1), 16–21.

Lasater, K. (2007). High-fidelity simulation and the development of clinical judgment: Students' experiences. *Journal of Nursing Education,* 46(6), 269–275.

Leigh, G.T. (2008). High-fidelity patient simulation and nursing students' self-efficacy: A review of the literature. *International Journal of Nursing Education Scholarship,* 5(1) Article 37.

Leigh, G., & Hurst H. (2008). We have a high-fidelity simulator, now what? Making the most of simulators. *International Journal of Nursing Education Scholarship,* 5(1), 1–9.

McCausland, L.L., Curran, C.C., & Cataldi, P. (2004). Use of a human simulator for undergraduate nurse education. *International Journal of Nursing Education Scholarship,* 1(1), Article 23, 1–17.

Mole, L.J., & McLafferty, I.H.R. (2004). Evaluating a simulated ward exercise for third year student nurses. *Nurse Education in Practice,* 4, 91–99.

Peteani, L.A. (2004). Enhancing clinical practice and education with high-fidelity human patient simulators. *Nurse Educator,* 29(1), 25–30.

Potts, N.L., & Mandleco, B.L. (2007). *Pediatric nursing care for children and their families.* (2nd ed). Clifton Park, NY: Delmar Cengage Learning.

Radhakrishnan, K., Roche, J.P., & Cunningham, H. (2007). Measuring clinical practice parameters with human patient simulation: A pilot study. *International Journal of Nursing Education Scholarship,* 4(1), 1–9.

Rauen, C.A. (2001). Using simulation to teach critical thinking skills. You can't just throw the book at them. *Critical Care Education,* 13(1), 93–103.

Rothgeb, M.K. (2008). Creating a nursing simulation laboratory: A literature review. *Journal of Nursing Education,* 47(11), 489–494.

Rush, K.L., Dyches, C.E., Waldrop, S., & Davis, A. (2008). Critical thinking among RN-to-BSN distance students participating in human patient simulation. *Journal of Nursing Education,* 47(11).

Rystedt, H., & Lindstrom, B. (2001). Introducing simulation technologies in nurse education: A nursing practice perspective. *Nurse Education in Practice,* 1, 134–141.

Schoening, A.M., Sittner, B.J., & Todd, M.J. (2006). Simulated clinical experience: Nursing students' perceptions and the educators' role. *Nurse Educator,* 31(6), 253–258.

Seropian, M. (2003). General concepts in full scale simulation: Getting started. *Anesthesia & Analgesia,* 97, 1695–1705.

Seropian, M.A., Brown, K., Gavilanes, J.S., & Driggers, B. (2004). Simulation: Not just a manikin. *Journal of Nursing Education,* 43(4), 164–169.

Seropian, M.A., Brown, K., Gavilanes, J.S., & Driggers, B. (2004). An approach to simulation program development. *Journal of Nursing Education,* 43(4), 170–174.

Thompson, T.L., & Bonnel, W.B. (2008). Integration of high-fidelity patient simulation in an undergraduate pharmacology course. *Journal of Nursing Education,* 47(11), 518–521.

Wilford, A., & Doyle, T. (2006). Integrating simulation training into the nursing curriculum. *British Journal of Nursing,* 15(17), 926–930.

Index

Page numbers followed by *f* indicate figures.